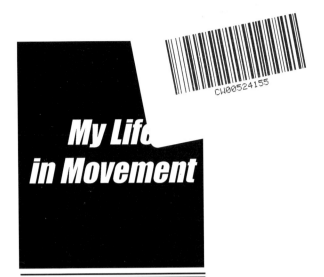

My Life in Movement

BY THE SAME AUTHOR

Margaret Morris Dancing, with Fred Daniels, London,
Kegan Paul, Trench & Trubner (1925).

The Notation of Movement, London, Kegan Paul,
Trench & Lubner (1928).

Skiing Exercises, with Hans Faulkner, London, Methuen (1934).

Maternity and Post Operative Exercises, with Sister M. Randell,
London, Heinemann (1936).

Tennis by Simple Exercises, with Suzanne Lenglen,
London, Heinemann (1937).

Basic Physical Training, London, Heinemann (1937).

My Galsworthy Story, London, Peter Owen (1967).

My Life in Movement, London, Peter Owen (1969).

Creation in Dance and Life, London, Peter Owen (1972).

The Art of J. D. Fergusson, Glasgow, Blackie & Son Ltd. (1974).

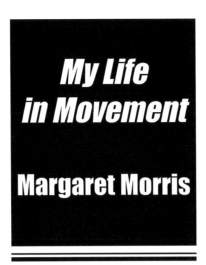

My Life in Movement

Margaret Morris

Illustrated with photographs and
the author's own drawings and diagrams.
Research and documentation
by Isabel Jeayes

© 1969/2003

Text © Margaret Morris 1969.

First published in Great Britain by Peter Owen Ltd, 1969.

This revised and updated edition published by
The International Association of MMM Ltd,
Garelochhead, Scotland, 2003.

British Library Cataloguing in Publication Data. A catalogue
record for this book is available from the British Library.

ISBN 0 9531034 1 2

Design and typeset by Bettany Press, London.

Printed by CLE Print Ltd, Huntingdon, Cambridgeshire.

*Margaret Morris Movement acknowledges with grateful thanks
financial contributions from the Nina Hosali Foundation and the
estate of the late Beryl Brooks, which have made this
new edition possible. Thanks are also due to those who
demonstrated their faith in the project by providing advance
subscriptions towards its publication.*

Dedicated to

ELIZABETH CAMERON

(*and to the not-so-young — who could be younger*)

*Elizabeth Cameron (née Ainsworth) was one of
my best dancers and has been teaching my work
for over fifty years, making it a record for the
longest consecutive teaching work of M.M.M.
So I salute her with deep affection and admiration.*

Contents

	PAGE
List of Illustrations	viii
Preface	xi
Foreword to New Edition	xiii
Part One: Growing Older	1
Part Two: Growing Younger	167
Afterword by Gillian Farenden	221
Bibliographical references	232
Index	233

LIST OF ILLUSTRATIONS

PAGE

Jim Hastie	xii
'Pastorale': A dance by Margaret Morris	xiv
Reciting programme, 1896	4-5
Margaret Morris reciting at the age of five	7
Royal Court Theatre programme	12
Margaret Morris with her first troupe	14
Gluck's 'Orpheus' at the Savoy Theatre, 1910	14
Programme designs for the early children's seasons	16
'Cinderella' at the Royal Court Theatre, 1912	18
Programme design by Margaret Morris	26
Penelope Spencer	29
Portrait of Margaret Morris by J.D. Fergusson	30
First Summer School, 1917	35
Third Summer School, 1919	35
Sketch of Juan-Les-Pins	37
Margaret Morris, Leslie Goossens and Betty Simpson at Eden Roc	38
Elizabeth Cameron high-jumping at Eden Roc, 1923	38
Opening of the Hôtel du Cap d'Antibes, 1870	40
Visitors to Eden Roc, 1924: George Bernard Shaw, Pablo Picasso, Marlene Dietrich	41
Margaret Morris at Cap d'Antibes, 1924	42
André Sella with Margaret Morris's pupils, 1923	45
Margaret Morris at her Club, 1921	49
Children with scoliosis doing M.M. Exercises	56
Drawing of Margaret Morris exercises by a disabled child	59
A page from The Notation of Movement	61
Children at Dr Rollier's clinic doing M.M. exercises on skis	70
Boys from Betteshanger School	74

Roland Harper demonstrating at the
London Training School, 1937   84
Illustrations from the prospectus of the
Basic Physical Training Association, 1938   85
Suzanne Lenglen and Margaret Morris   87
Jack Skinner demonstrating at Aldershot 1935   88
Jack Skinner and Elizabeth Cameron in
Dances at the Fortune Theatre, 1937   94-95
Celtic Ballet: 'Scottish Fantasia'   109
Celtic Ballet: 'Skye Boat Song'   109
'Barley Bree', 1954   112
'Corn Riggs', 1961   113
'The Deil's Awa', 1952   113
Celtic Ballet design   117
'Design and Action' performed for Scottish TV, 1959   119
Margaret Morris practising, 1965   135
Margaret Morris Notation: 1928 and 1969   149-150
Margaret Morris Notation: 1928 and 1969   152
Transition and Expression signs   155
Article for 'Donald of the Burthens'   163
Mental Attitude/Diet/Exercise   172
Opposition Movements   188
Anatomy of Breathing   192
Basic Breathing   192
Inspiration/Expiration   193
Basic Breathing: Lying   194
Basic Breathing: Standing   194
Anatomy of the Spine   195
Remedial spinal positions   196
Spinal movements   197
Pelvic and thoracic mobility exercises   197
Stretch to wake   199
Energising Exercise 1   201
Energising Exercise 2   203
Energising Exercise 3   205
Energising Exercise 4   207

(*continues over page*)

Invisible Exercise   208
Renewing Exercise   209
Armchair Exercises   210-11
Ironing out the spine   214
Hip rolling   215
Neck Exercise   216
Eye Mobility   218
Secret Exercise   219
Margaret Morris Movement display team
at the Royal Albert Hall, 1985   226
Beverley Currie, Jim Hastie and Janet Houselander
at the Canadian Summer School   231
Class at the 2002 Summer School,
Wall Hall, Hertfordshire   231

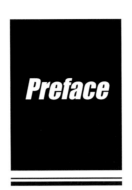

Preface

I AM SEVENTY-EIGHT YEARS OF AGE, and can honestly say I feel younger and better — although I don't claim to look younger! — than I did thirty years ago. As I am so often asked what I do and what I eat to make this possible, I think it is time I wrote a book about it. My personal 'routines' are the outcome of my whole 'Margaret Morris Movement' (M.M.M.), so I am giving an outline of the way this evolved before going on to detail more recent developments, which are the result of over fifty years' personal trial and error, and which I think show that it is possible to grow younger after fifty.

I am indebted to Dr Douglas Latto for taking time to read and advise me on the chapters dealing with anatomy, diet and exercise. Ivor Guest, the ballet historian, very kindly checked the chapters on ballet and modern dance.

Finally, I would like to pay tribute to our last, most generous benefactor, Herbert Ross, who made substantial contributions during our last years in Glasgow. It started by a friend telling him of my ambition to establish a Scottish National Ballet. He thought this should be done, and asked me to bring some boys and girls to dance in his garden at Cove. Their performance delighted him, and during tea he remarked, 'I believe you are short of funds,' and taking an old envelope from his pocket, he scribbled something on it, saying, 'Take this to my office.' It read, simply: 'Give Miss Morris £250. H.R.'

Margaret Morris, 1969

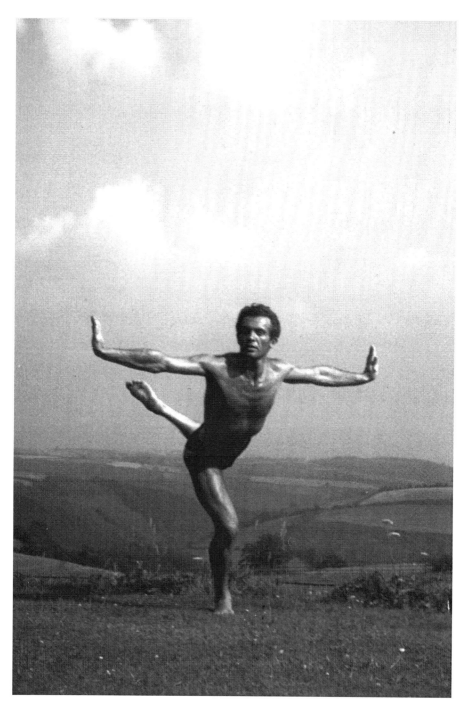

Jim Hastie. Photograph: Ruth Jeayes.

FOREWORD TO THE NEW EDITION

WHEN MARGARET MORRIS WROTE *My Life in Movement* in 1969, it marked the end of over 50 years of teaching her method. At that time the future looked a little bleak for Margaret Morris Movement; the full-time training schools had closed and the future seemed far from secure. However, the publication of the book brought her and her method to the attention of a wider audience. New training courses were set up, and suddenly things were in full swing once more.

With a new Board of Directors to support her, Summer Schools continued. *My Life in Movement* became a standard text book on the history of MMM for students training as teachers, as well as being eagerly read by those who had trained during the 50-year period. *My Life in Movement* also marked the beginning of the modern developments of MMM.

Sadly it has been out of print for many years, and it was a great ambition of mine to have it reprinted. Thanks to the generosity of those who had faith in the project, we are able to present this brand new edition of the work. There are some new photographs and an update chapter to bring MMM into the new century – alive and kicking!

Reading and re-reading her books during the course of preparing this work for reprinting, I am constantly struck by Margaret's words of wisdom and the importance of so many of the theories she put forward in earlier years which are thoroughly in tune with modern developments and thinking.

I think she would be pleased with it.

Jim Hastie
President and Artistic Director

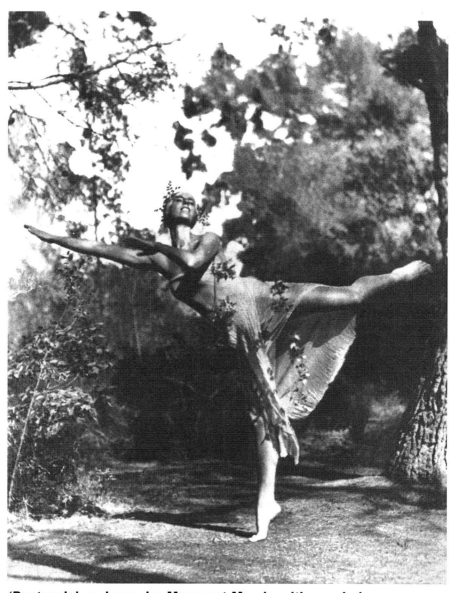

'Pastorale': a dance by Margaret Morris with music by
Stravinsky. Photograph: Fred Daniels.

PART 1
Growing Older

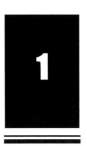

I WAS BORN IN LONDON IN 1891 of Welsh and Irish parents. My father was a painter and we went to live in France when I was only a few weeks old, so my first vivid memories are of France, and the beach at Boulogne, when I was about two and a half, with me running and jumping at the edge of the sea, my first free expression in movement! I remember even now the thrill of feeling myself a part of the sea, the sand and the wind. How wildly happy I was! I wanted it to go on and on, and I screamed with rage when I was carried up the beach and taken home.

I could not make the grown-ups understand what my discoveries meant to me, so I told my dolls about it, and showed them the shells and seaweed I had found, and how I had run and jumped over the small waves, and stretched up my arms to feel the wind. It seems my mother heard me talking to my dolls and watched my movements through the door, and this gave her the idea that I was born to be an actress or a dancer and she started to teach me La Fontaine's *Fables* and French poems. I loved reciting, and at three years old got engagements at parties, being stood on a grand piano, or big table.

Also at this time I gave the first indication of choreographic ability by collecting stones and shells and grouping them on the floor, moving them in formation, explaining that they were waves, fairies, etc. A few years later I did the same thing with squares of coloured paper, which gave me colour arrangements as well as formations, and then drawing the ground plans. When I was about five, we came to live in London. I spoke only French, but soon learned to recite in English as well as French and had engagements at big London receptions and country houses, often attended by Royalty.

Grosvenor Club.

BOND STREET.

-❄- SMOKING CONCERT -❄-

THURSDAY, 21st MAY, 1896.

AT 9.30 P.M. PRECISELY

PROGRAMME.

I. Miss JOSEPHINE SULLIVAN (Harpist)
"La Patrouille,"   -   -   *Hasselmans*
SELECTION from *Cavalleria Rusticana* - *Mascagni*

II. Miss LYLA KAVANAGH
"La Petite Parisienne,"   -   -
"Because I love thee so,"   -   -

III. Mr. ARTHUR DEANE
"Yeoman's Wedding Song,"   -   *Poniatowski*
"Beauties Eyes,"   *Tosti*

**IV. Miss MAISIE TURNER and
       Miss BELLA EDWARDS (Duettists)**
"Par une belle nuit,"   -   -   -   *Gounod*
   a. "I would that my love,"   -   *Mendelssohn*
   b. "La luna immobile,"   -   -   *Boito*

V. Miss BENITO LINDO
"Good Bye,"   -   -   -   -   *Tosti*
"To stay with you,"   -   -   *Hope Temple*

VI. Miss GERTRUDE LONSDALE
"A mother's love,"   -   -   *Hope Temple*
ARIA from *Samson and Delilah*   -   *Saint-Saëns*

VII. **Mr. AVALON COLLARD**
Song, - " ," -

VIII. **Signor BOROWSKI** (Violin)
" Berçeuse," - - - *Godard*
" Masun," - - - *Borowski*

IX. **Miss VERENA CHOLMLEY** (Character Song)
" I don't want to play in your yard," *H. W. Petrie*

X. **Messrs. BROUGHTON BLACK and AVALON COLLARD** (Duettists)
" The Rivals," - - *Black and Hastings*
" The Buttercup Duet," - - *Sullivan*

XI. **Madame ROSA FALTERRA**
{ *a.* " Thistle-Down," - -
{ *b.* " Mistress Rose," - - -
ARIA, " Non so più cosa son,"
(*Nozze di Figaro*) *Mozart*

XII. **Mr. BROUGHTON BLACK**
" Long ago in Alcala," - -

XIII. **Miss RUBY VERDI** (Danseuse, aged 12 years)

XIV. **Miss MARGARET MORRIS** (Recitations) *age 5*

XV. **Miss GWENNIE HASTO** (Comedienne and Danseuse)

XVI. **Miss EVA OSBORNE** (Plantation Songs)

XVII. **Miss ADA REEVES**
(From the Duke of York's Theatre, by kind permission of Mr. HORACE SEDGER).

XVIII. **Miss MARIE KEHREIN**
" Killarney," - - - *Balfe*
" When the heart is young," - - *Buck*

XIX. **Mr. CHARLES BERTRAM**
Will perform a few of his Wonderful Sleight-of-Hand Tricks.

I went to my first dancing classes when I was six, to a well-known teacher — Mrs Wordsworth. What impressed me most was her black satin dress, which had so many jet buttons down the front of the bodice that I could never manage to count them all.

My first professional stage engagement was in a pantomime at Plymouth when I was eight. I played first fairy, 'Little Twinkle Star', and also recited before a front drop. From there I joined the Ben Greet Shakespeare Company, and spent three years playing Puck, pages, and dancing.

Between tours, I had lessons with John d'Auban, ballet master at Drury Lane Theatre; he gave me the only lessons in ballet I ever had. I am grateful to him, for he put great emphasis on 'grace' and 'flow' of movement. It is difficult to believe, in this present age, how hide-bound the classical ballet was at the beginning of the century: d'Auban's methods were not approved of by the ballet purists.

I was quick and keen to learn but strongly resented the barre practice which of course I had to do. I found it unbearably boring. D'Auban was very patient and explained that it was essential to have a basic technique for the training of dancers, to which I agreed, but said, 'Why not create a new basic technique for those who don't want to be ballet dancers, but need a technique on natural freer lines, from which to develop a more creative type of dance and dramatic ballets.' Of course D'Auban said that nothing could ever replace the barre practice, to which, with the confidence of youth (I was only twelve) I replied, 'I will replace it, not for ballet, but as an alternative training for a freer type of dance.'

I started right away composing exercises, each with a definite objective — spring, balance etc, and I chose music for each that suggested the manner in which the exercise should be done — strong, light, smooth and so on. The way music was used in most ballet classes shocked me; only the tempo seemed to matter. From this time on I did no more ballet. My lessons had always been interrupted by tours, and now I decided I would only practice my own exercises, and compose dances.

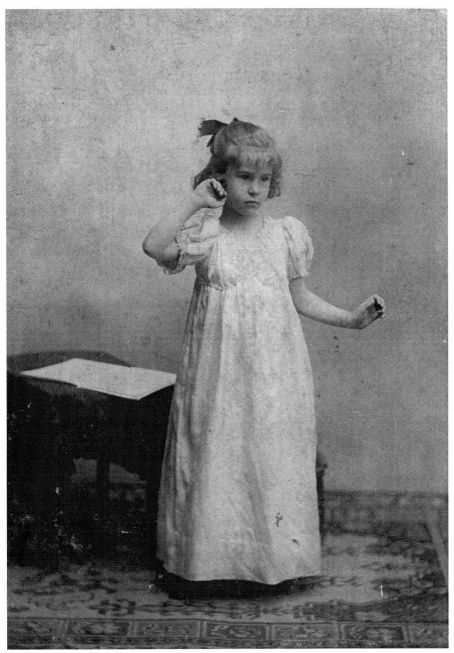

Margaret Morris reciting at the age of five.

Then followed a dreary period. I was too tall for children's parts, and too thin and immature for grown-up ones. Though I went on composing dances and exercises, I was conscious that I looked like a spider doing them, with my long thin arms and legs. At fourteen I felt my life was over.

Then, one day I put up my hair, borrowed a long skirt of my mother's, and went to see d'Auban, begging him to put me into the Drury Lane pantomime ballet. This he did, and although I had to go in the back row, not having enough obvious sex appeal for the front, it was wonderful just to be working in a theatre again. The girls of the ballet were a tough lot, but good-hearted and most generous with the little they earned. I got a liberal education into the seamy side of life from the experiences they related and the bawdy stories they told, but I had the good sense not to report these to my family. What did shock me however was the frying of kippers on the round wire guards over the flames of the gas brackets; newspapers were spread over the dressing-tables to catch the drips, but they did smell!

For a time I was happy, but when the pantomime season ended I was again in despair till I got into Frank Benson's company, playing ingénue parts and dancing. I was also to understudy Mrs Benson, and this thrilled me, for ever since I joined the Ben Greet Shakespeare Company at the age of nine, my great ambition had been to play Juliet, Ophelia and Lady Macbeth. I knew them all by heart, but it was not to be. Mrs Benson was very healthy and prided herself on not 'letting her public down', so she never missed a single show, carrying on even with a streaming cold or racking cough, while I stood by, vainly hoping she might collapse from the strain, and almost contemplated putting poison in her tea.

At the end of two years of playing Jessica, Sweet Anne Page, Phoebe etc, and realising that I was too young to graduate to second leads, I left. But they had been two very happy years. It was good experience, I made many friends, and had two proposals of marriage, which I firmly refused.

Benson was always friendly, and he asked me to arrange massed dances in the open for two pageants he was directing at Romsey and the Isle of Wight. This work was utterly frustrating, dealing with crowds of amateurs who could never manage to come together for rehearsals, and having to shout instructions through a mega-phone (no loudspeakers in those days) — dreadful! The only things that kept one sane were the endless amusing, even comic incidents; myself leading the War Maidens round the field astride a huge cart-horse (it was like straddling a dining-room table) wearing a helmet over a flaming red wig, blowing in the breeze; then the need to employ a team of men with shovels and buckets to rush on after each episode to remove the droppings from the many horses who galloped, shambled or merely stood around through almost every episode, until at the end of a solitary horseless scene, which ended with a procession of nuns, the shovel-and-bucket team rushed forward as usual, to be arrested by the megaphone-voice booming out: 'All right, boys! No need to clear up after the nuns!'

By now I had filled out and become more attractive, so I set to work in earnest on the technique I was evolving, and composed more dances based on it. A well-meaning family friend, wanting to bring my work before the public, most generously hired the Town Hall at Hampstead, where she lived, and arranged for me to give a recital there. But this charming, unworldly woman knew nothing of the necessity for publicity to draw an audience when presenting anything unusual. I knew it myself, of course, but my family had no money, and this kind friend was not really rich, so we could not ask her to do more than she had already offered to do.

To me the recital was a depressing affair. It was a matinée, and one could not shut out the daylight. I had worked for months on my programme of dances, giving interpretations of Bach, Scarlatti, Beethoven and Grieg. Musicians and artists who came were enthusiastic, but there were no press notices, so it really did nothing to advance my career. Soon after this (I think I was eighteen), I met Raymond Duncan (Isadora Duncan's brother), who was in London lecturing on the way of life of the ancient Greeks and on their dance and music. A friend of my mother's who admired my own dancing, and knew of the new dance technique I was trying to evolve, was taking a course with Duncan, and offered me his last two lessons, which I joyfully accepted.

From Duncan I learnt the six Greek positions and variations, copied from early Greek vases in certain museums. He explained that these positions, with their accentuated opposition of arms and legs, must have been the basis of the athletic training and the dance of the ancient Greeks. On doing them I realised this might well be true, for they use every muscle in the body and give wonderful body control and balance; and I decided at once to include them in my basic technique, with full acknowledgement to Raymond Duncan, and to make them form a part of every class. So in a way they have become the equivalent, in the M.M. technique, of the daily barre practice insisted on by the classical ballet.

I could not however agree with Duncan that these positions contained *all* that was necessary for the training of creative dancers. I wanted my technique to equip the dancer as completely as possible, while allowing the fullest personal freedom, so I included also certain movements of ballet origin, such as entrechats and arabesques.

Some of the first solos I composed and danced were interpretations of Grieg's 'Peer Gynt Suite'. (My 'Anitra's Dance' is taught as a class dance to this very day.) So when I heard that a Scottish woman, Isobel Pagan, was to put on her own translation of Ibsen's 'Peer Gynt' at the Little Theatre in London, I got in touch with her. I cannot remember how this came about, but someone must have introduced me, for I was always shy and incapable of forcing my way anywhere on my own. At all events she was charming, and delighted to let me compose and produce the dances for her play.

Miss Pagan's was the first full-length production of 'Peer Gynt' to be performed in England; and although I knew Greig's music well, I had never read the play, and I found that my solo to Anitra's dance, which was an interpretation of the music only, failed to fit the dramatic situation. Anitra was an Arab slave-girl, and it had to be an Eastern dance of seduction. I still don't think the music suggests this at all. It is very light and tripping, and I had used a lot of entrechats and springs, all of which had to be changed to snaky arm and voluptuous body movements, but I did my best to create the Eastern atmosphere required, for this was my first chance to work with a big group, except in pageants, and although the dancers were mostly amateurs and not trained in my technique, I enjoyed working with them, and I learnt a good deal from the experience.

In 1910 Gluck's 'Orpheus and Eurydice' was put on at the Savoy Theatre by a German opera star named Marie Brema who sang Orpheus, Viola Tree singing Eurydice. It was a friend of my aunt's, a Miss Schubert who was a direct descendant of the composer, who introduced me to Marie Brema, suggesting to her that my new technique, based largely on the dance of Ancient Greece, would be suitable for this opera. Marie Brema was delighted with the idea and gave me a free hand, even letting me design the costumes and scenery; she also advertised for dancers who wanted to train in the new Greek Dance technique. They came to me for a month before rehearsals. Among them was Ruby Ginner, who was quick to learn the Greek positions, and later started 'The Society of Greek Dance' in which she is still active. The only one of that group I am still in contact with is Norah Shone, who was only sixteen at that time when I started my school; she trained as a teacher and taught and danced for me for many years. She has a wonderful memory and still remembers the ballets I composed for 'Orpheus', though I myself have forgotten them.

This was my first big chance in a West End theatre, and I seem to have made the most of it. The *Daily Express* said: '....The triumph of the production is Miss Margaret Morris's dance of the Furies. Nothing like it has ever been seen on the London stage.'

It was on the stage of the Savoy Theatre, after the first performance, that I was introduced to John Galsworthy, and subsequently became friends with him and his wife Ada. I arranged the dances for a fantasy of his, 'The Little Dream', and

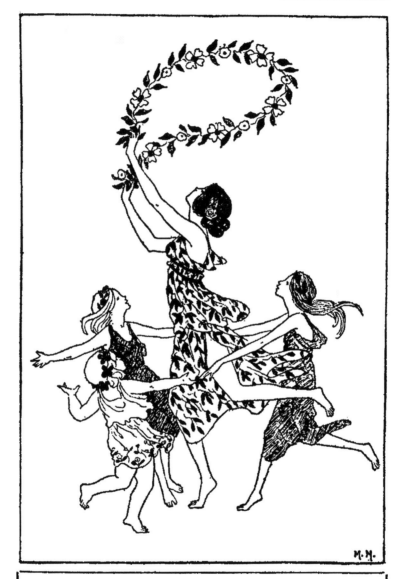

ROYAL COURT
THEATRE, SLOANE SQUARE, S.W.

MARGARET MORRIS
AND HER DANCING CHILDREN

later acted with Dennis Eadie and Gladys Cooper in his play, *The Pigeon*. Working with John Galsworthy was my first big emotional experience, for I fell deeply in love with him, and although our relationship remained entirely innocent, it had a profound and lasting effect on my life and my work. But I have already told this story in my last book.[1]

It is not generally known that it was John Galsworthy who was responsible for my starting a school at all. My father had no private income. Being a painter, his earnings were very precarious, so we could not possibly have paid additional rent for even one room for a school. When I trained the dancers for 'Orpheus' and 'The Little Dream', a room was provided for my classes: but such hurried, short-term methods were most unsatisfactory. I had to take either quite untrained people, or dancers who had been taught classical ballet and turned their feet out all the time. In either case one could not get very good results with only a few weeks' training, as John and Ada Galsworthy realised: so they undertook to finance a modest start if I could find a suitable room, which I did over a milk-shop only a few minutes' walk from our flat at the top of St Martin's Lane. I arranged an audition there, and John helped me choose the six children who formed my first troupe, which was called 'Margaret Morris and her Dancing Children'.

At that time my whole interest was in the theatre, and I still saw myself as a great actress as well as a dancer. It never occurred to me that teaching and the running of the school would absorb more and more of my time, and how my interest in the health and remedial applications of my work would grow. But as it was John's idea that I should start a school, and as he helped me repeatedly over the first three years of its existence, I feel that although he could never be the father of my child, I can claim him as the father of my Movement, which is my only child.

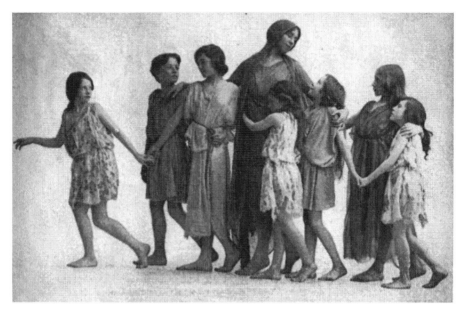

Margaret Morris with the first children chosen to train by John Galsworthy.

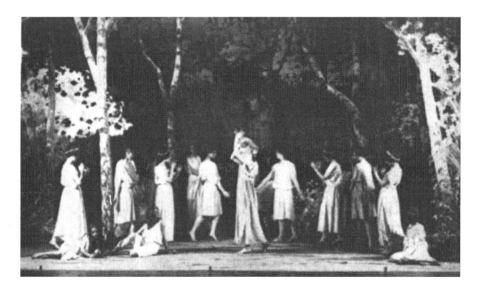

**Gluck's 'Orpheus' at the Savoy Theatre, 1910.
Margaret Morris is at the centre of the stage.**

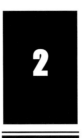

2

IN A FEW MONTHS THE M.M. INFANT had outgrown its cot, and I managed to find a really large room in a stained-glass factory in Endell Street, close by Seven Dials. At this time, besides holding classes for children and adults during the day, I was playing Water in Maeterlinck's 'Blue Bird' at the Haymarket Theatre. Meanwhile my school was growing all the time, and in a year the Endell Street premises also had become inadequate, mainly for lack of dressing rooms. There was only a curtained alcove which also contained the piano, so I could never have male and female pupils at the same time.

It happened that one of my most enthusiastic pupils was a Greek scholar, Gerald Warre-Cornish, and he took it upon himself to find better premises for the school, if possible at a place where we could start a small theatre as well. These he eventually found, but to my great sorrow they were in Chelsea. I was extremely unhappy to leave my beloved Theatreland, and I resisted at first, but had to give way because the Chelsea premises were so suitable — a first-floor room 100 feet long, with direct access to Flood Street at the corner of King's Road, quite near the Town Hall. It was obvious, even in those days that premises as big as the Chelsea ones would cost a fortune in the West End.

Gerald thought they were just what we needed, and when I pointed out that the rent (which I think was £100 a year) was more than double what we paid in Endell Street, he said at once that he would pay the whole of the first year's rent to give us a start, and would continue to help if necessary. So what could I do but gratefully accept, and early in 1912 we moved the school

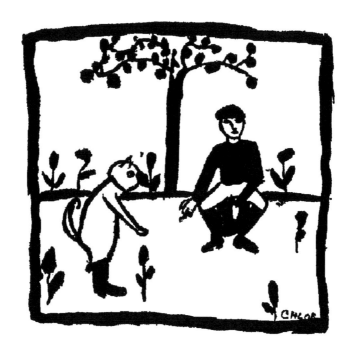

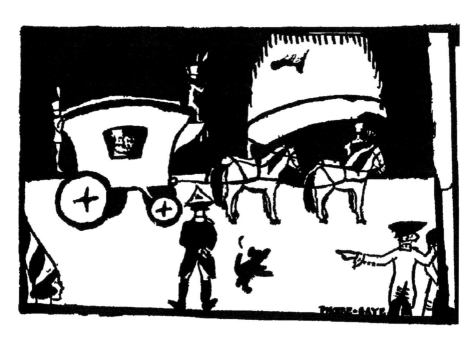

Programme designs for the early children's seasons.

to Chelsea. I decided I would give a season at the Royal Court Theatre, and include Galsworthy's 'Little Dream', because none of the West End managements would put it on: and from October to November 1912 I did so. The programme also included a ballet written for me by Maurice Hewlitt and some original dances.

By this time we had put raised seating into the school theatre, and the classes were held on the stage. At Christmas 1912 I gave my first Children's Season. We put on 'Cinderella', the title role being played by Kathleen Dillon (now Mrs Angus Morrison), with Iris Rowe as a tiny fairy queen. These two were in my very first troupe.

All the performers were children, and the programme design was by Phoebe Gaye, aged twelve. We applied to the LCC for a temporary theatre licence, so that we could take money at the doors. This was eventually granted, but we had to fix lighted EXIT signs of the regulation size as used at the Coliseum and Olympia.

By chance there were two exits, with broad stone steps and double doors, but we had to fit them with safety push-bars. This expenditure proved well worthwhile, however, for these Children's Seasons became a regular feature for many years to come. They were always well filled, though as our seating could only accommodate an audience of under 150, we barely covered our expenses even when playing to capacity.

I am almost certain that mine was the first of the really small theatres in London, and that these Christmas shows were the first *for* children *by* children. We used to let the theatre sometimes to other experimental theatre groups, professional and amateur; John Gielgud told me not long ago that he made his stage debut at the age of nine in an amateur production at my theatre.

Early in 1913, soon after the close of our first Christmas season, I had the opportunity of taking a troupe to Paris, to dance at the Marigny Theatre in the Champs Elysées. I felt this was a great opportunity: I had not been to Paris since I was a small child and I longed to see it again. An old friend of my

My Life in Movement

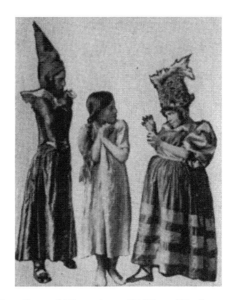

'Cinderella' at the Court Theatre, 1912, with Angela and Hermione Baddeley as the Ugly Sisters (above); Phoebe Gay and Gwendoline Thoms as the Prince and Cinderella (below).

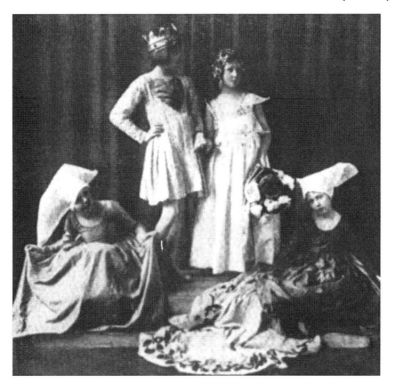

father's, who agreed we ought to go, gave me the money for the fares, but — as it has been all my life, though so many friends have helped me — there was no margin to spend on publicity, or to pay an impresario. So we crept into Paris and out again, and though our few performances were well received, we did not reach the big Paris public. The possibilities of my new technique were, however, recognised by a few artists and musicians, among them J. D. Fergusson, the Scottish painter, who greatly influenced my whole Movement and later became my husband: so for me the trip was momentous in its consequences.

My first meeting with Fergusson was characteristic. I presented myself at his studio — 83 Notre Dame des Champs — at four in the afternoon, bearing a letter of introduction from an old friend of his, Holbrook Jackson, who was Editor of *Today*, a progressive magazine of that time. Seeing no bell I knocked rather timidly on the door, which was immediately opened just far enough to allow a dripping black head to appear. 'Excuse me,' it said, 'but I am having my bath, will you please come back in half an hour?' Which of course I did, and was then most courteously received by Fergusson, wearing French workman's blue cotton trousers and a blue sailor's jersey; his hair was still wet and curly, and there was an aroma of carbolic soap. I think I lost my heart to him then, though I did not realise it until much later, as I was still acutely unhappy over the complete frustration of the love between John Galsworthy and myself, which I still believe could have enriched not only our personal lives, but the creative work we were both doing.

Fergusson was charming and kind at that first meeting, as he was throughout the forty-seven years I knew him. He made tea in a round Japanese teapot that figures in several of his paintings — I have a small one by me now. The decoration of his studio enchanted me, it was so light and gay; white walls, furniture painted white or a flesh-coloured pink, with vivid coloured cushions and bowls of brightly painted dried oranges. Some people said it looked more like a ladies' boudoir than a studio, but there was certainly nothing cissy about Fergusson; he was just completely unconventional when he wanted to be.

At Antibes in the summer he always wore a broadbrimmed peasant woman's hat, because it gave more shade than a man's; he said it was only men lacking in virility who were afraid of being thought effeminate. On the other hand he always dressed very conventionally when he went out because he did not want to look like an artist. He even wore a bowler hat and a well-cut overcoat, but when they wore out he took to a soft hat and a trench coat because they cost less, and any money he made he spent on paints. All his life he put his painting before everything else, yet he always found time to help anyone who wanted to break away from academic art, and he would never accept fees for his teaching.

At that first meeting he promised to teach me to paint — and he did. He said he would come and see me dance and interest his friends — and he did. He devoted whole days to taking me to art galleries and exhibitions, and this certainly was not because he was interested in me as a woman. The first time he made drawings of me he said, 'You have a perfectly proportioned figure but there is not enough upholstery!' Obviously, from the sex angle, I just did not exist, but he admired my courage in breaking away from the classical ballet and creating a new technique, and he thought I might become a painter and he wanted to help me, and of course it was his idea that the study of form and colour should be an essential part of a dancer's training.

Fergusson's philosophy was one of joy, though he had been one of the angry young men of his decade — angry at the obvious injustices of life, but he believed that however hard the struggle for existence, creation in art should emerge from realisation of intense happiness, and not from misery and hardships. When he was worried or depressed he did not paint at all, sometimes for months on end, for fear it should get into his painting. Some people thought he went too far in putting his painting before all else in his life, but he was always perfectly frank about it. He told me after I had only met him a few times that he had no intention of ever producing any children. He believed that all genuine spontaneous art was an act of creation, as much as the act of making love; but if children were produced the artist must either sacrifice his children to his art, or his art to his children, neither of which was he prepared to do.

In 1905 he had gone to live in Paris, which certainly proved his spiritual home. The Scottish Academy of that period dominated the art life of Edinburgh, they were solidly conservative, and even rejected the paintings of Peploe. Pictures by Fergusson that were considered quite outrageous in Edinburgh, were at once accepted by the Salon D'Automne in Paris, hung, and several sold on the first day. He was made a Sociétaire du Salon d'Automne in 1909; he was accepted and welcomed by the modern artists including Matisse, Derain, Segonzac, Braque and Picasso.

Many society women wanted him to paint them, but though he loved painting good-looking women, he would not accept commissions, or invitations from society hostesses. He insisted on keeping his independence and only painting what — and when — he wanted; most people thought he must have a private income, but this was not the case. He was often very poor, but he never borrowed money; he lived on porridge for lunch, and onion and potato soup for dinner, with an occasional night out when he met his friends at a cheap restaurant in Montparnasse, and invariably ordered a tournedos. He was gloriously happy; the Paris tradespeople were interested in artists, his laundress mended his clothes without being asked, and only added a few sous to the bill. He always said that Paris was the best place to be poor in; painters, writers and musicians could meet at a café and talk for hours over a cup of coffee. Most evenings Fergusson walked to the Dôme or l'Avenue on the boulevard Montparnasse to meet his friends. Sometimes they walked the boulevards arguing fiercely for whole nights on end; but Fergusson never quarrelled with anyone, people he did not like he avoided, so he was known and respected by many, had a few staunch friends, and made no enemies.

Fergusson was a tremendous admirer of the Diaghilev Russian Ballet, with its wonderful combination of music, décor, costumes and choreography, all designed by great artists: but he had never liked the point work or more conventional postures of the classical ballet, and when he saw the ease of movement of my pupils, and their freedom of expression, he had a vision of a production with décor, costumes and music equal to those of Diaghilev's ballet, but with dancers trained on a much freer technique. This was my vision too, but one that has yet to be realised.

Fergusson convinced me that an understanding of painting and design was essential to dancers who wanted to produce creative and original work. He also led me to share his enthusiasm for Indian and Cambodian art, taking me repeatedly to the Trocadéro Museum, with its wonderful collection of ancient Eastern sculpture. I made endless sketches of their dancing figures, and this influence can be seen in many of my exercises, hitherto based purely on the Greek tradition. As soon as I got back to London I started classes in painting and design along Fergusson's lines, and made these compulsory for all those of my pupils who were training for the stage.

Very early in my teaching career I realised the need for a practical method of recording dances and exercises as music is recorded. On enquiry, I found that there had been several in the past, and I was lent the manual of one of these entitled *Playford's Dancing Master*: but none had proved practical for theatre-dance, particularly not in the recording of new departures in dance technique, so I felt it was up to me to do something about this. Raymond Duncan had a simple way of indicating the placing of the arms in his Greek positions, but he had no signs for the legs and feet: so I worked out easy-to-write symbols for steps forward, back, sideways etc, and demonstrated with children, showing how my pupils could read and perform the positions I wrote on the blackboard. Over the years I gradually evolved this method and a book on the subject was published in 1928.[2]

This system of dance notation interested the composer Rutland Boughton, whom someone brought to my theatre about this time. He appreciated to the full what I was trying to do in the world of dance by establishing a freer technique than that of the classical ballet, and encouraging creation in all the related arts. We found we had much in common, and I was especially thrilled with his idea of 'dancing scenery', just the kind of experiment I wanted to do: so when he asked me to cooperate in his Summer School at Bournemouth in August 1913, I gratefully accepted. I took a group of my pupils, and we slept in tents, which I enjoyed very much, and ran classes and rehearsed all day long.

The school ran for three weeks, culminating in public performances at the Bournemouth Winter Gardens, with Dan Godfrey conducting his Symphony Orchestra. The 'dancing scenery' was for the first scene of Act II of Boughton's opera, 'The Birth of Arthur': the male chorus were the walls of Tintagel Castle, and the females, led by my dancers, were the sea surrounding it and the waves breaking on the castle walls. My pupils and I also did a selection of our original dances, and a short ballet to music by Rameau, called 'Phyllis and Corydon'.

During those three weeks I was also going over the music for the dances in 'The Immortal Hour' with Boughton, who had just finished writing it. It was to be performed at the Glastonbury Festival in the summer of 1914. Unfortunately I never produced those dances, for I was in the South of France when the war started, and was delayed there. But I sent several of my pupils to Glastonbury, including Penelope Spencer who produced the dances for 'The Immortal Hour' at the festival, and re-did them in 1922 for Barry Jackson's London production.

Rutland Boughton composed the music especially for our second children's production at Christmas 1913 of 'Snow White and the Seven Little Dwarfs'. I played the Wicked Queen and Eleanor Elder (who later started the first Travelling Theatre) was the Butcher, the rest of the cast being children. Iris Rowe was Snow White, Kathleen Dillon the Prince, and Angela Baddeley gave a really remarkable performance as the First Dwarf. They all wore masks, with big noses, but the expression Angela got into that mask of hers was quite incredible. It seemed to be always changing with the angle of her head and the movements of her hands, and somehow she made that comic little dwarf a most moving and lovable character, who quite stole the show.

In the autumn of 1914, after the outbreak of World War I, Fergusson came to live in London. He took a great interest in my school, and for several years he took the painting classes personally. This was wonderful, because the pupils' enthusiasm grew rapidly, and some of them were soon doing really interesting paintings and designing costumes for their dances in the Christmas programmes, and later for the Margaret Morris Club, which Fergusson and I started in 1915.

In the early days of M.M.M. my mother did all the secretarial work and the accounts, but when we moved to Chelsea and started theatre shows and the Club, she could not cope with it all, as she was cook-housekeeper for the family and also caterer for my Club, for which she made wonderful soups. So we got a secretary, and how lucky we were: Mildred Stokes was with us for years, a devoted and efficient worker, seeing us through the most difficult times, keeping our creditors at bay — for we were always hard up and behind with the rent and taxes — but through it all she was cheerful and helpful. Since her retirement she has lived in Ilfracombe, but still takes a lively interest in M.M.M.

The idea of starting a Club came to us because Fergusson missed the café life of the impecunious artists in Paris, and having enjoyed it myself for several months, I realised the terrible lack of it in London. In Paris you could talk all night on one cup of coffee, or drink as much as you wanted and could afford, each paying your own bill: and you could meet all kinds of interesting people — painters, writers, actors and musicians. London, on the other hand, was completely dead in the evenings as far as popular refreshment was concerned: so unless you could afford to entertain and give parties, or join clubs, there was no way of meeting people.

It is difficult for the young of today to realise what it was like in 1914 and even many years later, when apart from the West End theatre and restaurants, the glittering night-life of London depended on private entertaining and went on behind the closed doors of wealthy private houses. After a few tea-shops closed, you could not even buy a cup of tea or coffee. Nowadays there are countless coffee- and milk-bars as well as licensed bars, and even pubs have become respectable. Women can and do go to them freely. When I was young it was unthinkable for any woman with the slightest pretensions to respectability to be seen going into a public house.

So the Margaret Morris Club was started; it was to be a centre for free discussion, and for presenting original creative work in the arts. It was not a licensed club — we served tea, coffee and lemonade: but it became a meeting-place for painters, writers and musicians, not only from Chelsea, but from many other parts of London.

We had three meetings a month. On the 7th there was a performance of original dances, sometimes set to poems or songs, with costumes, and sometimes with décor as well, designed and painted by the dancers. The 14th was always a free-for-all discussion, and we persuaded most interesting speakers to open these, choosing any subject they liked: only politics and religion were barred. The 21st was a social evening with ballroom dancing, and in this too we encouraged people to improvise, so there was never a dull moment. Sometimes, Eugene Goossens, Cyril Scott or Constant Lambert would sit down and improvise on the piano and generate a real excitement.

The Club opened during the First World War and became very popular with officers of the French Army and Navy when they were in London, as well as with our own. Some members of the Diplomatic Corps also attended, and many theatre people. It was an extraordinarily interesting mixture, and any kind of dress was allowed; beautiful evening clothes, uniforms, slacks and sweaters, all mingling happily together.

It was a wonderful education for our students to meet such artists as Augustus John, Epstein and Wadsworth, writers like Katharine Mansfield, Middleton Murry, Ezra Pound, and the writer-painter, Wyndham Lewis. Two other colourful and interesting artists who attended regularly were Lett Haines and Cedric Morris. Lett looked very like a faun in those days, and I loved dancing with him, for he improvised wonderfully, and we

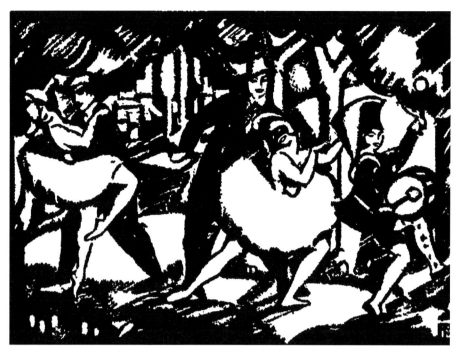

Programme design by Margaret Morris for a ballet produced at the club.

used to leap around and between the other dancers, sometimes to the dismay of the more sedate couples. Cedric is now Sir Cedric Morris, Bart., and a keen horticulturist, well known for a new type of iris he has grown. To Fergusson and me they were simply artists, and our very good friends. Many years ago Cedric and Lett started an art school together near Hadley in Suffolk, which we thought an excellent idea; but in spite of repeated invitations we never managed to visit them there, though I still hope to see their school some day.

The Scottish architect, Charles Rennie Mackintosh, with his wife Margaret, were frequent visitors at my Club, and Fergus and I often dined with them at their studio in Glebe Place, or met them at the Blue Cockatoo on the Embankment. They had left Scotland, completely discouraged by the lack of appreciation of Mackintosh's work in his own country. In Germany, Austria, Holland and elsewhere he had been hailed as the pioneer of modern architecture, which he certainly was, and toasted at banquets as 'the Master': but though he built the Art School in Glasgow, a most wonderful building of international fame, it found no favour with the local authorities and no further important commissions were forthcoming. So he decided to settle in London and the South of France and to devote himself to painting.

I recent met the son of William Davidson for whom Mackintosh had designed a now famous house, Windyhill. This man had inherited from his father a batch of letters from Mackintosh to his wife, written from Port Vendres, and several of them mention Fergusson. I have permission to quote the following passage:

> Your letter is very interesting because you say that 'Fergie' liked my pictures. I don't think that artistically there is any other artist I would like to please better than Fergusson and Margaret Morris also.

I feel all this is relevant to my story because while he was in London he designed a theatre for me, feeling the converted hall in Flood Street was unworthy of me and my work. The designs and plans are set forth in a book by Howarth, together with his designs for a block of studios. I knew the theatre would not materialise, for I never had any sufficiently wealthy backers: but the flats were a practical proposition because there was such a need for them that they were all let in advance. However, when the designs were submitted to the appropriate body they were turned down immediately. Because there were no decorations on the walls, the authorities said the building would look like a factory. They agreed to pass the plans if bunches of fruit or flowers were added but Mackintosh of course refused to do this and the studios were never built.

The year that I am writing this, 1968, is the centenary of Mackintosh's birth. This has been celebrated by a notable Memorial Exhibition during the Edinburgh Festival, sponsored by the Scottish Arts Council. It was planned and carried out by Professor A. McLaren Young of the University of Glasgow. It was shown in the Victoria and Albert Museum, London, and abroad in Darnstadt and Zürich. The European showings are most appropriate, for it was on the Continent that the value of Mackintosh's work was first recognised, long before it was appreciated in Britain.

Angus Morrison, already a brilliant pianist though still in his early teens, played for most of our Club shows, and a lot of interesting and original work was produced, for I was lucky in having several exceptionally gifted pupils, who have since made names for themselves. Besides Angela Baddeley, I had her sisters Muriel and Hermione, and Elsa Lanchester was with me for two years. When she came she was more Greek than I had ever been, wearing only handwoven Greek tunics, with bare feet and sandals in all weathers. She had a mass of flaming red curly hair with a Greek fillet round her brow. When she left me she started a cabaret, the 'Cave of Harmony', and later met and married Charles Laughton, with whom she worked in films and in the theatre.

Rosalind Iden, who later married Donald Wolfit and is now Lady Wolfit, was an excellent pupil and danced in many of my shows: but I felt her interest was always more on the dramatic side than in pure dance, and this has been borne out in her acting career.

Joan Lawson was a creative dancer as a child, but soon after she left me she turned to classical ballet, and has since become quite an authority on 'the dance'. For twenty years she was critic for the *Dancing Times*, and she is now on the staff of the Royal Ballet School.

Penelope Spencer, who had arranged the dances for 'The Immortal Hour', created many original solos: and after she left me she continued to do some very interesting work. In 1919 she joined the Glastonbury Players as dance director and choreographer. She was solo dancer in several operatic productions at Covent Garden, and arranged the movements for the first production of Shaw's *Saint Joan*, with Sybil Thorndike. She is now married, with three grown-up sons.

Another outstanding pupil was Blanche Ostrehan, who came

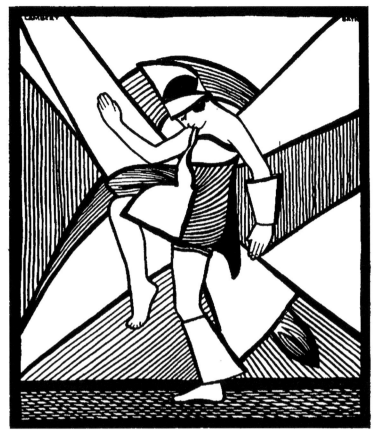

**Penelope Spencer, one of Margaret Morris's
most successful pupils.**

to me in 1916. From a child she had longed to be a dancer, and I feel that in a way I failed her because, though she did become a wonderful dancer in her own particular, rather oriental style, which had a quality of magic, and though she danced in 'Hassan' at His Majesty's in London, and under Fokine in New York, yet as far as *I* was concerned, she finished up as my best teacher of Maternity Exercises, at which she was particularly successful. She followed me in this work at Stonefield Maternity Home in Blackheath, which was run by a Dr Pink and a Dr White! When the war started the Home was evacuated to Wookey Hole in Somerset, at the invitation of Mrs Elsa Barker-Mill, whose first child was born at Stonefield, where she had done my exercises: and Blanche continued teaching these Maternity Exercises for several years after the war ended. I wanted her to join me in Scotland in the 1950s, and help me train the Celtic Ballet there, but she felt that if she herself could no longer dance she would rather do something quite different. This she did, taking a variety of jobs, in the mountains behind the Riviera, in England breeding Siamese cats, and finally in a home for disabled people with learning difficulties. She has now retired, but is still one of my greatest friends.

It was around 1916, too, that the first man to want to train as a professional dancer came to me, Rupert Doone. He did not stay very long, but we gave him his basic training, and he took a prominent part as dancer and choreographer in the emerging English ballet of the late 'twenties.

Many other of my pupils did interesting work, but it is impossible to mention them all. I felt I was training a new race of dancers, who created dances and designed costumes besides performing, in my Club. I myself was having great personal success in my solos, 'The Golden Idol' to Ravel's arrangement of Debussy's 'Le Poisson d'Or', Debussy, and Dvorak's 'Humoresque', though only before a limited Club audience: but I

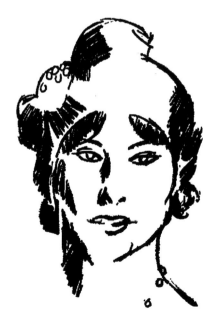

Portrait of Miss Margaret Morris
by John Duncan Fergusson.

was also doing short tours with a small company to the larger towns, the Manchester audiences being always a special joy. I took a mixed programme of dance and drama, the last because I longed so much to go on acting, but choice of plays was difficult. It was hard to find actors who could dance, and dancers who could act, and at that time I had no men whom I had trained myself.

Meanwhile I was always searching for new forms of expression in dance and design. I loved Beethoven's Seventh Symphony, and when someone told me it had been called 'the Dancing Symphony' I said I would make this name come true. I designed different costumes for each movement, for by this time I had gone beyond the purely Greek tunics and draperies for every production, though I still used them when suitable. Some people did not like my costumes, but they would look quite modern now.

I put on 'the Dancing Symphony' first at my club, although the stage was too small and we could only have a piano accompaniment, so it gave me little satisfaction. For years I had dreamed of dancing with big orchestras, and of doing choreography for great symphonies, not merely using them to accompany some ballet for which they were never intended, but trying to give a visualisation of the music in movement and design. So, remembering how I had enjoyed producing the dances for 'The Birth of Arthur' , I wrote to Dan Godfrey at Bournemouth, telling him about my 'Dancing Symphony'. He was at once interested, and offered me an engagement at the Bournemouth Winter Gardens, telling me to bring my Company and present the Seventh Symphony, with a programme of dances and ballets.

The Bournemouth presentation was a great success, and it was here that the Symphony was seen by a little-known agent called Briggs, who had the idea of booking us at other Winter Gardens, where there were big orchestras who could play it. This he did, fixing some quite well-paid engagements at Harrogate and Bath, as well as return bookings at Bournemouth. This was the first time I had been able to enjoy dancing with large orchestras, but though we were very successful in the provinces, Briggs never managed to get us an engagement in London. Unfortunately for us he was not among the leading agents, but he certainly persevered. He suggested booking a smaller group of six or eight, doing twenty minutes of short dances at certain cinemas which were actually converted theatres, so that they had a stage behind the screen and whose clientele liked a live show between two films.

Accordingly I prepared a twenty-minute programme of short dances, keeping to our standard of first-class music, but with plenty of variety in the dances themselves, some of them with mime, some abstract patterns, and some humorous. When Briggs got us a date at a big cinema in Brighton I was delighted, because I have the happiest recollections of Brighton in my touring days as a child-actress in melodramas, and later in Shakespeare.

At the first performance I sat in front, full of apprehension, to gauge the reactions of the audience; but, to my relief and astonishment, our act was well received even at the first house; it was twice nightly. I believed if I could keep a small group touring, it would mean work and experience for my dancers.

But an unfortunate thing happened; our agent Briggs, who could not have been more than forty, died very suddenly — how or why I never knew. It was a great blow to us. He was a very ordinary, inconspicuous young man, but he got us jobs and we never had any disagreements. No other agent took any interest in us. The only opportunities for dancers were in musical comedy, pantomime or variety, and agents would say they could only book troupes like the Tiller Girls, or dancing acts of tap or pure acrobatics. They would not even look at anything that departed from these conventions. Yet only a year or two before, Maud Allen had caused a sensation and danced to packed houses, just because she was doing something different. The general public only comes to see the new and the unusual if it has enormous advance publicity and is presented as something sensational.

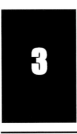

IN 1916 I BECAME RESTIVE. I longed to get away from London, and smell the country and the sea again. My family could never afford holidays, but touring had given me changes of scene and had often taken me to seaside towns. I never wanted to go anywhere without working, but I liked my work to take me to nice places, as Rutland Boughton's pre-war Summer School at Bournemouth did. There we worked incessantly, but in lovely surroundings, and I thought how wonderful it would be during the summer months to rent a house in some place by the sea, where we could dance and paint in the open, and bathe and lie in the sun; and in the evenings we could walk, talk and dance, and perhaps have outdoor performances.

In those days, when the idea of summer schools and intensive courses had not yet taken hold, it was easy to find houses or schools to rent. My first two Summer Schools were held in 1917 and 1918 at Combe Martin, North Devon. Many pupils and friends came, and we all enjoyed ourselves despite the much too frequent rain. For the third summer, the first after the war ended, we went to Harlech at the invitation of a wealthy man named George Davison, who lived there. Eugene Goossens had brought him to my Chelsea Club, and he was so delighted with the natural grace and free movement of my pupils that he proposed we hold our next Summer School at Harlech where he had built a beautiful house, called Wernfaur, which had a very large hall and lovely gardens. He suggested that if we could find accommodation for our pupils in the village, we could hold all our classes in his gardens, or, if it was wet, in the big hall, where in the evenings we could have discussions, concerts and dances. I was delighted at this generous offer, and in the summer of 1919 our school was held at Harlech.

G.D., as he liked to be called, was a remarkable man. For many years he had been Chairman of the London branch of the Eastman Kodak Company, having launched the Kodak firm in England, but he had lately retired and taken to adopting children. When I first met him he had adopted nine. His greatest interest, apart from this one of giving neglected or unwanted children a wonderful start in life, was music, and he invited the most distinguished musicians to come to Wernfaur to work or to rest. So during our two Summer Schools there we met some extremely interesting people, mostly from the musical world. Among the musicians I remember were Granville Bantock, Cyril Scott, Arnold Bax, Harriet Cohen, and of course Eugene Goossens whom I knew already as he had helped me in my little Chelsea theatre.

By a strange coincidence, I recently read Eugene Goossen's fascinating autobiography* and I found in it an account of my school at Harlech, and of Fergus' painting classes, which I feel may be of interest here, so I will quote from pp.138-9:

> To complete the artistic colony at Harlech, there arrived at that time Margaret Morris and her School of Dance. This consisted of a group of young women and men whose plastic posing and 'self-expressing' calisthenics in short Grecian tunics were the pride and joy of the locality. 'Meg' Morris and her assistants held classes on the seashore and in the courtyard of 'Wernfaur', imparting an Attic flavour to Harlech that surprised and occasionally shocked, the elders of the town. . .
>
> John Duncan Fergusson, eminent Scottish painter, a source of inspiration and help to the Morris clan, came along as usual to supervise the rather Cezanne-ish efforts of the School in its afternoon painting work, which took place out of doors, unless the weather was too bad; the students adored

*Eugene Goossens, *Overture and Beginners* (Methuen, 1951).

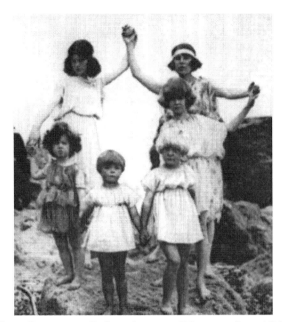

First Summer School, near Ilfracombe, 1917.

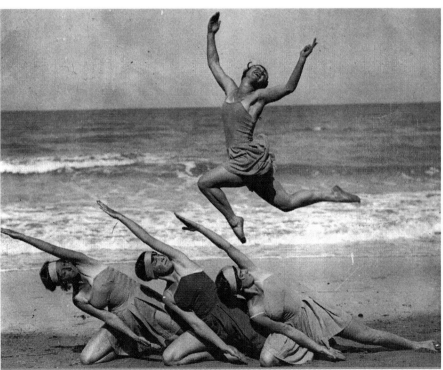

Third Summer School, at Harlech, 1919.

'Fergus' for his patience and efficiency and his faculty for linking up in his lectures the twin plasticities of paint and body movement. The rhythmic improvisations of the dance — in which Meg and her pupils excelled — he translated into terms of colour and brush strokes, so that, at Harlech, the two arts were synonymous in theory and practice. I helped to add a smattering of music to the curriculum by an occasional lecture on rhythm and form.

Everything about our Harlech Summer School was perfect — *except the weather!* It rained and rained. So we decided to try France the following year and we took the Château des Deux Rives at Dinard, on a promontory overlooking the sea on two sides. But the weather was not much better than it had been in Devon or Wales, and as George Davison had been so good to us we went back to Harlech in 1921: but once again the weather was against us.

A year later we tried Pourville, near Dieppe, a charming place and a memorable Summer School, for many artists, musicians and writers joined us, including a delightful American poetess, Edna St Vincent Millay, who read her poems to us. But here again the weather was very variable: and I, who knew what real summer was like in the South of France, longed to organise a Summer School down there.

The chance to do this came about in an unexpected way. G.D.'s youngest child Doreen (then only about two years old), was lovely to look at but very delicate, and the winters in Wales did not suit her, so Fergusson persuaded him to take her to the South of France. They went to an hotel in Juan-les-Pins, and G.D. wrote, delighted, saying: 'But the sun always shines here! I shall never return to England.' He bought a house, the Villa Gotte, next to the Casino — (it is still there, but turned into flats) — and invited Fergus and myself to spend Christmas of 1921 with them there. It was wonderful. I remember we had Christmas dinner out of doors in the sun.

G.D. told us he wanted to find a suitable property, big enough to house all the adopted children, and of course it must have a

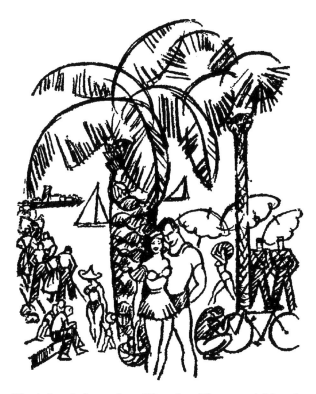

Sketch of Juan-les-Pins by Margaret Morris.

private bathing-place. In 1912, while cycling round the Cap, Fergusson had noticed a large half-built house next to the Hotel du Cap: and on asking about it he learnt that the building had been started by King Leopold of Belgium for his mistress, Cléo de Merode. But when the walls had reached the height of the first floor, the King was told he could not build any higher, as the house would cut the beam of the Phare, the lighthouse in the middle of the Cap, whose light perpetually swings over it. So the building was abandoned, and it had stood there for sixty years, till trees grew in the stately rooms.

Fergusson told G.D. about it, and I remember vividly the excitement of exploring it for the first time. There were extensive grounds, with pinewoods going down to the rocks, and a long sea frontage of deep water on the Baie d'Argent, facing due south. We were all enchanted with the place, and G.D. at once decided he would buy it. We clambered among the bushes and

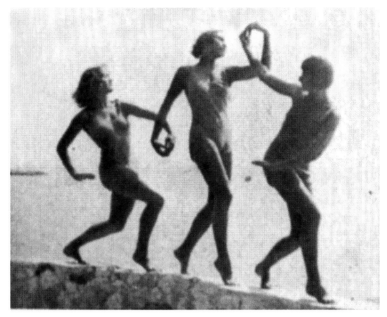

Margaret Morris, Leslie Goossens and Betty Simpson at Eden Roc.

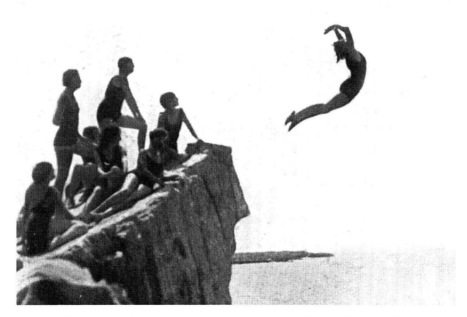

Elizabeth Cameron high jumping at Eden Roc, 1923.

trees growing inside the solid stone walls that still bore white chisel marks, looking as if they had just been made: the air was pure and clean. The window openings were immensely high, about 12 feet, and the building itself was about 200 feet long, divided into six or seven large rooms.

Ever since I was a child I have loved making plans of houses, which I am able to memorise after just one visit. I saw at once that the number of rooms that were needed could be achieved by putting in an extra floor at each end of the building, making two floors of low-ceilinged rooms at either end, while leaving the full height for the reception rooms in the middle. I drew a rough plan, which G.D. at once approved, and got a French architect to act upon.

By the summer of 1921 the building was well under way, but I stayed again at Villa Gotte, running straight out of my bedroom on to the sands to bathe. Juan-les-Pins was still completely deserted and the Casino was offered me for sale as a school, for a mere song! Alas, I hadn't got a song! But I arranged to rent the Hôtel Beau Site, between the Garoupe Beach and the Hôtel du Cap, as our Summer School for 1923. At the same time I arranged for the necessary staff to be engaged. There were no labour problems in those days, everyone on the coast being unemployed in the summer.

The school was a great success. In those days it *never* rained on the Riviera during June, July and August, and pupils and friends from England and northern France came flocking down there, eager for guaranteed sunshine. One could travel from London to Antibes third-class return for £7 10s 0d, not too comfortably I must admit, but the young didn't mind.

The day after we arrived, old Mr Sella, owner of the Hôtel du Cap, called on me and, after some preliminary courtesies, said he believed I had with me some very lovely young girls. I wondered what was coming, until he explained that he believed he might be able to initiate a Summer Season at Eden Roc, something that had never been tried hitherto. The Hôtel du Cap was closed, but he invited me to hold our classes in the grounds under the pine trees, and to bring my pupils to bathe every day

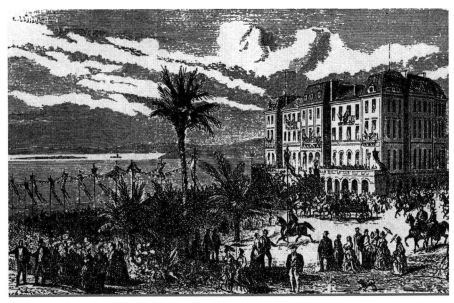

Opening of the Hôtel du Cap d'Antibes, 1870.

at Eden Roc, saying he would organise some international publicity. We needed no urging to carry out this programme. We covered ourselves with oil and sunbathed on the flat roof of the Eden Roc Pavilion, and the press were invited to photograph my pupils diving off the rocks and dancing in the woods. The pictures appeared in *Vogue*, the *Tatler*, the *Graphic*, and in corresponding European and American publications.

By this time G.D. had sold Villa Gotte, he had sent for all the furniture from his house in Wales together with all the adopted children, and had moved into his new home, which he called Le Château des Enfants (now La Résidence du Cap). Once again he opened his doors to my pupils and our friends, always making us welcome, as he had done at Harlech.

Mr Sella told us he was going to make 1924 the start of the Summer Season, when he would open the Hôtel du Cap and invite a few chosen guests, among them Picasso with his first wife, a Russian ballerina, the Comte de Beaumont, and Scott Fitzgerald. He insisted that we must come back the following year for it. He put at our disposal three empty cottages quite near the hotel, putting in camp beds and odd bits of furniture. My

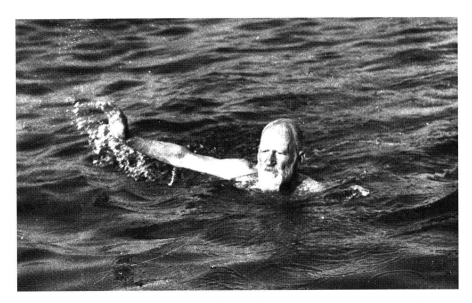

George Bernard Shaw, one of the visitors to Eden Roc in 1924.

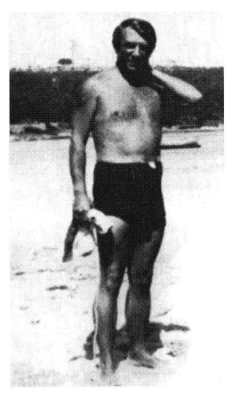

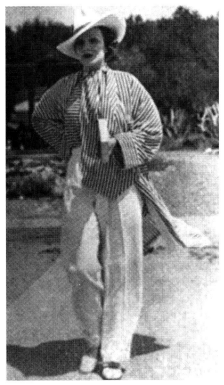

Pablo Picasso at Eden Roc.   **Marlene Dietrich at Eden Roc.**

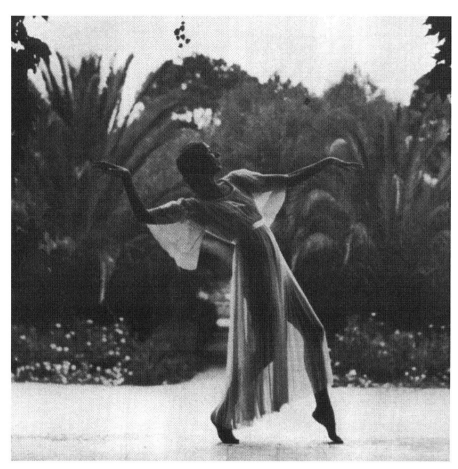

Margaret Morris dancing at Cap d'Antibes, 1924.

girls camped there most happily and Mr Sella was charming to them. He used to go to market in Antibes in a big lorry, and he would take some of them along, so that they could get fruit and vegetables at his special trade prices.

Nineteen-twenty-four was a great year. We all had to work very hard, but we enjoyed every minute, giving performances at night in the hotel grounds. Mr Sella took endless trouble, installing raised seating and hiding spotlights in the trees, thus enabling us to achieve some wonderful effects. The shows were well advertised, and we got an audience from all along the coast. When the French fleet was at Juan-les-Pins, Mr Sella gave dances and invited the naval officers to them, so my girls had a gay time. Some of them still remember the number of ice-creams they consumed on these occasions, for Mr Sella was a generous provider.

My principal teacher and dancer at the Antibes Summer School was Lois Hutton. She was one of the best teachers I ever had, and although she was only with me for four years, she made important contributions to the Movement. She had a good figure, an excellent brain, and was a fine gymnast, being employed as senior teacher of Physical Education and Games at Roedean School, when she came to my Summer School at Combe Martin in 1918. She was enchanted with the freedom of movement and the encouragement of original ideas in dancing and painting, and at once decided to give up her good, safe job at Roedean in order to study with me. In an incredibly short time she had learnt my technique and assimilated my ideas, as well as Fergusson's on painting.

She became responsible for planning and systematising the teachers' training, and introduced the study of Anatomy and Physiology, subjects on which she had already lectured. She also helped me greatly with my *Notation of Movement*, and was invaluable in all the teaching aspects of my work. Yet it was the dancing and theatre side that had attracted her. Although she composed most effective dances and was one of the best dancers in my Company, she found, as I did, that when running a school, one's energies are given more and more to making others dance, and less and less to dancing oneself.

So Lois decided not to return to England, but to settle in France with one of my French pupils, Hélène Vanel, an attractive dancer of great intelligence who is now a lecturer on art at the Louvre. Together they started a tiny theatre right inside the little hill town of St Paul, near Vence, and called themselves 'Les Danseuses de St Paul'. The room only held an audience of forty, and was lit at first only with oil lamps and electric torches: but their shows were so well attended that they often had to repeat the performance after midnight. Lois Hutton rode the Cossacks' horses when they came to St Paul, married a Russian, stayed in France all through the Second World War and later organised musical and dramatic recitals at her little theatre, and befriended all the needy cats of the neighbourhood.

Meanwhile the Summer Season at the Cap was becoming increasingly successful, spreading all along the coast, and more and more English and American visitors flocked to the South of France each year. Statesmen from many countries, business tycoons, film stars and aristocrats were to be found sunning themselves right through the hottest summer months on Eden Roc. The Duke of Windsor, when he was Prince of Wales, often bathed there. I remember he passed me on the steps one day, wearing a pair of slacks held up by a piece of string, and I heard him say to a friend: 'Why bother with a belt? String does just as well.' So string became 'the thing' at Eden Roc!

Now all the world has heard of this Côte d'Azur paradise, and knows that it has the most wonderful deep-water bathing imaginable, but since it has become so fashionable, it has also become expensive. For the next two or three years I held a small Summer School at Antibes, though we had them in England as well: but eventually the Riviera became too dear during the once-neglected summer months. Meanwhile I had established a branch of my Movement at Cannes, which was run with great success by one of my pupils, Avril Gilmore, until the beginning of the Second World War.

For years now, the Hôtel du Cap and Eden Roc have been under the direction of André Sella, the son of old Mr Sella, who started the Summer Season. In 1923 André was a very young man, but he took a lively interest in our work, as can be seen from the snapshot taken when he posed for fun with a group of my girls in the hotel grounds. André Sella is now known to hundreds of people all over the world as the most considerate and charming host, always planning new comforts and enjoyments for his guests. But in spite of the international fame of his hotel, he never forgets what my dancers contributed to the launching of the Summer Season at the Cap d'Antibes. For many years, he has made me an honorary member of the Eden Roc Club and when I go there he and his family entertain me charmingly.

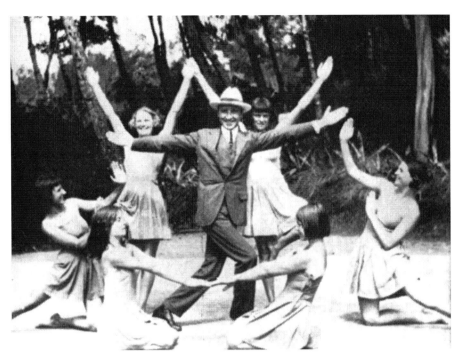

André Sella, proprietor of the Hôtel du Cap d'Antibes, with Margaret Morris's pupils, 1923.

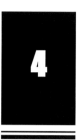

In 1917, THOUGH MY AIM WAS STILL to train dancers for the theatre, I could not but notice, and many parents pointed out, the remarkable improvement in my pupils' health and appearance: and I realise now that this must have been the beginning of my interest in the health and remedial possibilities of my Movement. It was also the parents who were largely responsible for my starting a school for general education. Many of them were dissatisfied with the ordinary schools, and regretted that their children could only come to my classes after five in the evening. Having escaped all conventional education myself, and never having missed it, I had very strong views on the subject. I admit it is useful to be able to spell and to add, neither of which I can do, but I believed then — and still believe — that the education of boys as well as girls should consist, up to the age of twelve, largely of languages, taught orally, and the arts. After that age, children can be made to realise that subjects they may find dull and difficult are necessary to fit them for their future careers, and they apply themselves much more readily, and learn quicker.

At that time, there were no educational schools that specialised in dancing, or indeed in any of the arts, which were regarded as 'extras': so I decided that I must start my own Educational School.

In 1918 I was living with my mother and my aunt at 1 Glebe Place, Chelsea, where I had the School office and wardrobe. The rent we paid was only £50 a year for the whole house. The wardrobe department was in the basement, where hundreds of costumes were made over the years by one of the most charming and competent people I have ever known, Mrs Shone.

She was of Irish extraction, and the mother of my pupil Norah Shone, whom I have already mentioned. Mrs Shone worked all day, and often far into the night in that front basement room, making elaborate costumes and fantastic head-dresses from my scribbled designs. She also made my own clothes, even my coats and hats. I rank her with Fred Daniels as one of my greatest benefactors.

The office was on the ground floor, and my aunt, Miss Maundrell, had the first-floor front room, where she conducted the day school. She was a really remarkable teacher, educated in France like my mother. For many years she taught French at Heathfield School, Ascot, having started doing so in Queen's Gate, where the school began. Though a strict teacher, she was adored by her pupils. I had a letter from one of them barely a month ago, asking if I could find a photograph of her. My mother took the Drama Classes at Heathfield for many years, and produced the plays at the end-of-term performances, sometimes taking me with her to play the principal part. I felt very professional and important, and I loved being with the children of my own age, but they seemed much younger to me and I was glad I had never been to school. The performances were always a tremendous success.

Of course, it was impossible to put my ideas on education into practice adequately in one room, so I started looking for a suitable house, and presently found one, a light and airy building at the corner of Cranley Gardens and Fulham Road. I engaged fully qualified teachers for the morning work, the afternoons being given up to dancing, painting, modelling and music.

Among my first pupils were Phoebe and Freda Gaye, who were already training at my dancing school. Phoebe became a successful novelist, and at a very early age Assistant Editor of *Time and Tide*. Freda had a distinguished career as an actress, and is now Editor of *Who's Who in the Theatre*.

The school ran for several years, but as usual I had started with no capital to back me, and the salaries of qualified teachers were higher than I had expected. Our running costs went up, and it often happened that the children I wanted to accept could not pay the full fees, and I would make a reduction; so eventually, we had to give up, much to the regret of parents and pupils. Quite recently I had two letters from married women who had attended my school, telling me how much they felt they owed to the start in life it gave them.

The Children's Christmas Seasons continued to be a regular event. One of the most successful of these productions was 'Jack and the Beanstalk' in 1922, in which Elizabeth Ainsworth (to whom this book is dedicated) played the leading part of Jack. Eliza, as she is generally known, came to me as a young child, attending the outside children's classes: but she was so obviously talented that we soon took her in as a boarder, so that she could do the professional training. She was undoubtedly one of my best and quickest pupils, and in record time reached the highest standard 'Emerald Green', and became a principal dancer in all our shows. She also composed several exercises, which I included in our technique. She is an exceptionally good teacher of Dance Composition and Improvisation, and has contributed several methods of Group Improvisation. She tells me I gave her children's classes to take when she was only fifteen, and as she is still teaching I am sure she must hold the record of the longest consecutive teaching of M.M.M.

One of my pupils of whom I am very proud is Phyllis Calvert. Although she gave up dancing for acting, as a child she showed exceptional ability in both, and my mother, who took the acting classes and produced the children's plays, was enchanted with her. Phyllis was a very small child when she first came to me, entirely on her own initiative, some time during 1922. She and her sister Vera used to creep up the long straight stairs, which led from the entrance in Flood Street right on to our classroom-stage. One day I noticed a flaming red-gold head (Phyllis) and a paler gold one (Vera) peeping over the top step. I called to them, but they disappeared, scuttling away downstairs and out of the building. Next day, however, they came back, and I managed to speak to them, asking if they would like to learn to dance. They were speechless, but their faces lit up, so I told them to ask their mother to come and talk to me, and this she did. She was a

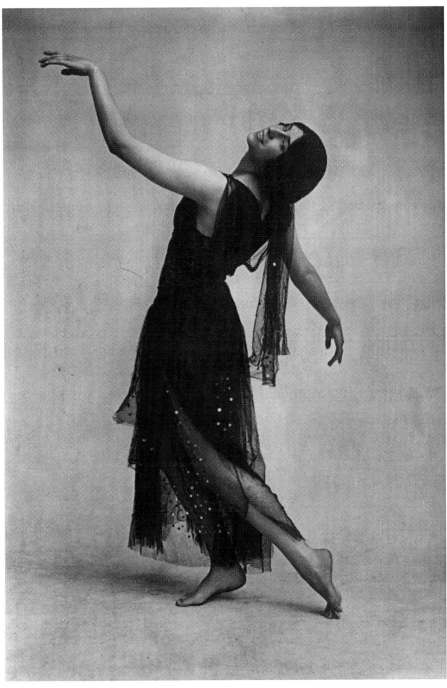

Margaret Morris at her Chelsea Club, 1921.

charming woman, always helpful and cooperative, which cannot be said of all parents.

Phyllis and Vera were soon enrolled for both dancing and acting, and each of them was successfully launched, in due course, on a professional career. But Vera never really took to the stage, and after leaving me she soon gave it up.

I remember Phyllis especially in *The Princess and the Swineherd*, a Hans Andersen story dramatised by my mother. She was the most adorable Princess, combining personal charm with the arrogance of manner necessary to the part. We also did scenes from *Alice in Wonderland*, in which Phyllis played the Dormouse and understudied Alice. One evening a London pea-souper fog descended, unknown nowadays, and Alice failed to appear: so Phyllis played the part at the shortest possible notice, with perfect confidence and most attractively. I have followed her acting career with lively interest, admiring her performances in many films, *Fanny by Gaslight* and *Kipps* among them: but I especially enjoyed her stage appearance as Peter Pan, which I loved. The way she moved did me credit!

Nineteen-twenty-two is also memorable for my meeting with the American dancers Ruth St Denis and Ted Shawn, who came that year to the London Coliseum and had a great success. I went to see them many times and thought they were wonderful. I was especially thrilled because they did original dances and no classical ballet. Though I cannot remember just how we met, I have the most vivid recollection of their coming to visit my school in Chelsea and watching my classes, and of what a help their admiration and encouragement were to me at that time. Also the fact that they were such a success in a Music Hall programme proved that a freer type of dance than the conventional ballet could have a popular appeal.

Several times over the years Ted Shawn invited me to come and teach my Movement and dance at his famous Summer School and Theatre at Jacob's Pillow, in the Berkshire Hills of New England, USA. But it was thirty-two years before I got to Jacob's Pillow, taking with me the first Scottish Ballet Company to visit America. This story, however, belongs to a later chapter.

About this time someone gave me a book on Hatha yogi, which impressed me very much. I kept it by me for years, and studied it with great attention, and it has had a profound influence on my work to this day. But it was only after Lois Hutton interested me in physiology that I became convinced of the supreme importance of breathing for both physical and mental well-being, and realised that it was absurd to put one breathing exercises in a long table of exercises, as though you could stop breathing for the rest of them. It should be obvious that breathing must be synchronised with every single exercise, so that the air is taken in on movements that expand the lungs and facilitate inspiration, and expelled when the body is doubled up, or the lungs compressed in any way, to assist expiration.

In Hathi yogi there are several different methods of breathing, each with a specific aim. It seemed to me that the one called 'The Complete Breath' was by far the most comprehensive, and the most suitable for my purpose, so I adopted it, while always acknowledging its origin. I made it the basis of all the exercises, eventually renaming it 'Basic Breathing'. Needless to say I had great difficulty in getting my dancing students to accept this innovation. They sensed, and of course they were right, that my increasing interest in the health and remedial possibilities of my work would draw me away from the purely aesthetic and theatre side. Inevitably my ambition of a dance company of my own gave place to a wider vision to include all humanity. The theatre and my own dancing were always uppermost in my mind, yet I felt I had to develop the remedial side, which I envisaged so clearly as part of an aesthetic whole, and it came to me that this movement that seemed to be evolving through me — even though it was not what I had at first intended — could be adapted for people of any age, even to those with grave physical impairments.

I realised that the more normal you could make people feel, the more normal they would become. They could not grow a missing arm or leg, but the more they could take part in normal physical activities, the happier they would be.

Many years later, I gave a big public demonstration in

Edinburgh, and I had a group of badly disabled boys aged 15 to 16 in the demonstration. Everyone was amazed that they were willing to take part, but on the contrary they were delighted to appear, and made the most ingenious use of their callipers and crutches as part of the designs, when forming groups. Afterwards they gathered round me, excitedly thanking me for a wonderful evening; and one of the boys said, 'You know, Miss, you are the first person to understand *we want to move!*'

All this time I was still training children and students for the theatre, and the Club was successful. I had composed many more exercises and incorporated some devised by my teachers, for I always tried to draw out the talents of my pupils, not to impose mine on them. The exercises were now graduated into ten standards, from the most natural and easy to the most complex and difficult. Then I suddenly had the idea of naming the standards by different colours, the students to wear tunics of the colour of the standard they were learning. Of course, I arranged the colours in my order of preference. At the bottom was White, for a new student is inevitably colourless, and the order then progressed upwards as follows: Yellow, Orange, Red, Pink, Crimson, Mauve, Blue and finally my favourite, Emerald Green.

The next step was to design a special tunic. Greek tunics hid too many faults of posture and depended too much on how they were put on; they could look wonderful, or they could look hellish. I designed a tunic with a tightly fitting bodice to the hip-line, elastic shoulder straps to allow freedom of movement and cut very low at the back to show the positions of the shoulder blades, and a short pleated divided skirt, so they could turn cartwheels or do hand-stands without showing their trunks. (Now of course this is unnecessary, as you can show almost everything without criticism.) Forty years ago my tunics were considered far too scanty; now they seem unnecessarily decent, and bright colours are the vogue. Thank heavens for that.

I see now what a hindrance it is to success to be too versatile: but when I was young, though I had no conventional religious beliefs, I had the firm conviction that if I always did only what I believed to be right, in the end I must succeed, and I felt it *must* be right to follow up every new idea that came to me. But I have learned to my sorrow, it is one thing to have a wonderful vision, but quite another to find the means wherewith to carry it out, and from this time I have been torn between my two great interests, Art and Healing: yet I still believe they should be united.

The remedial side of my work just seemed to be forced on me: people brought me children with lack of co-ordination, flat feet etc. There was a young girl who had had polio very badly and it had left her with a severe curvature of the spine and very weak legs (she wore callipers); she had had Swedish remedial exercises and hated them and refused to do any more; she told me she never felt she made any progress. I was not surprised, because the Swedish system consists largely of giving 'resisted movements' to work the weak muscles. Theoretically it is sound, but terribly frustrating to the patient, because every effort they make is resisted; they are merely told to try more and more, but they know they can't win, so there is never any sense of achievement.

I decided I would start from the opposite point of view, and give my patients only the movements they could do to begin with even though this did nothing for the weak muscles, so that they got the feel of enjoying moving, to music of course. Gradually I introduced movements for the weakened muscles, and as these were part of an exercise they wanted to learn, they made every effort to do the difficult movement, and little by little it would improve, till they usually achieved it, because I had established the possibility of success in their minds. I really did achieve some quite wonderful results. It took time, but my patients were never bored, and some went on joyfully for years.

I believe that all healing and corrective work should be approached with the eye of the artist, the creator. All great doctors and surgeons are artists at heart, and many do actually paint; but this point of view does not usually extend to the lesser branches of the profession, though there are of course notable exceptions. Nationally the physiotherapy side of medicine is my great interest, for there it is possible actually to use the point of view of the artist. Because all exercises can be made good to look at and interesting to perform, I don't think any patient should be asked to do ugly-looking movements, for I still believe that good cannot come out of bad, and also if a patient can enjoy a treatment, he is halfway on the road to recovery.

In 1925, I gave my first demonstration for doctors, at the suggestion of the father of one of my pupils. The father was a distinguished ear specialist who for two years had opposed his daughter taking the teacher's training, but who eventually became so convinced of the value of the work I was doing that he said I must make it known to the medical profession. His daughter was Betty Simpson, who eventually became my second-in-command. She was an excellent dancer and painter and a most wonderful all-round teacher and leader, with unbounded energy and enthusiasm. Dr Simpson made me a list of doctors he thought might be interested. We sent out about a hundred invitations, but on his advice kept it to the profession, not inviting the wives. To my surprise at least fifty must have come, for the Little Theatre was more than half full.

I don't think I have ever been more nervous than when I faced those rows of solemn men, with only one or two women among them. I told them frankly I had had no medical training, but for over ten years had studied the effect of my exercises on pupils, children and adults. I explained my ideas, which I have already recounted, and then pupils demonstrated the yogi breathing I used, the Greek positions, my basic exercises for balance, mobility etc. Then one or two disabled children showed how the normal exercises could be adapted to their needs, and also how they could take part in the aesthetic side of dance composition and improvisation to music. I ended by saying it was my hope that these experiments of mine might be developed and made use of on a big scale.

We were warmly applauded and the curtains were being drawn together when suddenly a man in the audience stood up: all heads turned towards him, and there was a hushed silence. He was a short, rather thick-set man, with white hair and a bristly white moustache. Of course, I had no idea who this man could be, but learned afterwards, he was Sir Robert Jones of Liverpool, accounted the leading orthopaedic surgeon in Britain. He delivered a wonderful speech — it made such a deep impression on me I can't forget it; he started by saying he did not know me and had never heard of me until he had received my invitation to this demonstration. He had come because he felt it was his duty to investigate any suggestions offered to help the disabled, but he had expected to be bored and unimpressed.

On the contrary, he said, he had found the whole demonstration quite enthralling, and was completely converted to my 'aesthetic approach' to exercise for the disabled. He had come prepared to criticise severely a layman's alleged contribution to orthopaedics, so he felt obliged to stand up and say that he could find nothing wrong with my arguments; every exercise I showed was medically sound, and based on logical reasoning. He respected that I made no claim to any medical knowledge, but he said he would have no hesitation in entrusting patients to me; in fact he had one in mind he would like me to start treating at once. He hoped other orthopaedists would make use of what I had to offer them. Then Sir Robert shook me warmly by the hand, and many others crowded round me, Mr Elmslie, Mr Bristow, Dr Murray Levick and many others, asking me to start classes in their hospitals or take their patients. There was far more enthusiasm than I had dared to hope for; I was joyful, for I felt that the great urge I had to spread my Movement beyond the limits of the theatre was going to be justified, and for a time it looked as if it really was to be so.

Sister Randell, head of the Physiotherapy Department at St Thomas's Hospital, asked me to take a class for her students, and she also formed a class of Sisters which she herself attended most enthusiastically. Mr Elmslie, orthopaedic surgeon at St Bartholomew's Hospital, started a class for children with scoliosis (abnormal curvature of the spine), which he often watched; he even suggested a special posture exercise to correct lordosis (hollow back) and I put it in our regular list so that it is still used. As a result, I evolved special exercises to

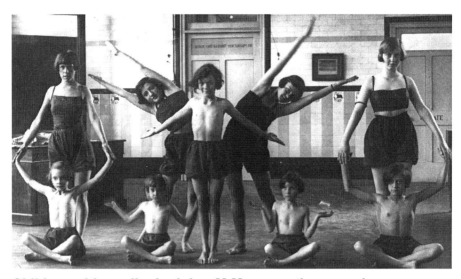

Children with scoliosis doing M.M. corrective exercises.

correct the various curves and I always gave deep breathing in corrective positions to stretch the contracted side. Of course physiotherapists were already doing this, but what was different about my method was that I approached the subject as an artist — putting the corrective positions into an aesthetic exercise. The children were correcting their deformities while making a pattern and they delighted in doing this because it was fun to be part of a group that was good to look at, and could be admired if they did it well. It was not just a boring exercise to do them good. In this way, I found that interest can be maintained indefinitely if the teacher has imagination, because there are always more exciting and more difficult exercises to learn. Normal breathing and mobility exercises are given as well as corrective ones, and when the children have learned their own special corrective positions, they are encouraged to compose groups themselves, and also to improvise to music. Music is of the greatest importance to keep the interest up over a long period, as to get abnormalities corrected repetition is essential.

Also as a result of the demonstration to doctors, Dr Murray Levick asked me to demonstrate at the Heritage Craft Schools for Cripples (as it was called in those days), Chailey, how I would handle a class of badly disabled children, and to meet Mrs

Kimmins, the founder, a great pioneer in the care of disabled people. She was an amazing person, full of energy and drive, and I feel privileged to have met her.

I went to Chailey for the first time enthusiastic and hopeful, but when I saw the group assembled on the lawn for me to teach, I was dismayed. I had never seen such badly disabled children. I was quite horrified, but realised at once I must not show my horror. How thankful I was that my long theatre training made me able to act the part of someone used to dealing with deformities, and therefore able to look at them and treat them as normal human beings. Half the class was carried and put on chairs, others hobbled out on callipers and crutches, and those who could walk were minus an arm, or both arms, or had withered useless ones.

I don't think I have ever felt so frightened. I had a double audience: Mrs Kimmins, the matron, the medical and many of the nursing staff were in rows behind me, and facing me were about forty disabled children gazing at me with expectant, wondering eyes. I took a deep breath and told them I was going to teach them the same exercises my other classes practised, but as they all had some difficulty in moving, some would do the arm movements and some the legs. I got them all moving — the sitting ones doing arm movements, the standing ones leg movements and walking round the chairs.

Then I tried to interest them in breathing. I explained we all had to breathe to keep alive and breathing was certainly one thing they could learn to do as well as people with no impairments at all. After that I asked the helpers to put the sitting ones in two groups on either side, some sitting on the ground just in front of those on chairs, the walkers standing at each side so that they could see what the other group was doing. I pointed out that the arm movements in the middle, and the leg movements at either side looked very nice, and I showed them how the ones sitting on the ground, by putting their arms above their heads, could make patterns with those sitting on the chairs. They became quite excited and I told them that if they worked hard, they would all dance with some part of their bodies.

The children had obviously enjoyed their first class and were asking when I could come again. Everyone seemed delighted; Mrs Kimmins was enthusiastic and indeed became one of my most staunch supporters.

I took the first two or three classes, and then passed them on to Betty Simpson, my second-in-command, and she proved herself wonderful at dealing with all kinds of disabled people. She had more patience than I, and was full of ingenious ideas for using crutches and wheel chairs as part of a design. A few years later we gave a matinée in aid of the Chailey Homes at the Savoy Theatre, and Betty Simpson designed and produced a ballet called 'The Enchanted Garden' in which all the Chailey classes took part. This was something unique. Betty had designed costumes to hide all the deformities; those who had to sit or stand were trees and flowers, and used their arms; those who could use their legs were rabbits or ducks, some were butterflies, with wings extended on thin sticks. The children were enchanted and at the end of the ballet, people crowded on to the stage to tell the children how good they were and how well they looked. One little girl called out to her mother 'Mummy, Mummy, the doctor said I'd never walk — but now I can *dance*!

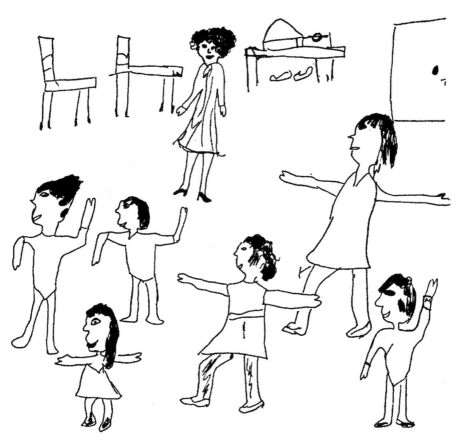

Drawing of Margaret Morris exercises by a disabled child.

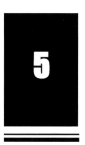

DURING THE NEXT TWO YEARS I was inevitably absorbed for a time in the remedial application of my work and could give less attention to the school and the theatre, which I left more and more to my teachers, keeping my contact with the artistic side of my Movement mainly through the Club, which went on as before. It was wonderful to find leading doctors and surgeons who had confidence in me and sent me patients. Some started classes in their own houses for their children and those of their friends.

Meanwhile I was also working on my book, *The Notation of Movement*, which I had been evolving since 1913, and which, as I have mentioned, was published in 1928 by Kegan Paul. This came about through C. K. Ogden, who created 'Basic English'. He had a first-class brain, and would talk for hours on almost any subject. He died some years ago, and I miss those discussions with him. He ran a magazine called *Psyche*, and edited a series of small books for Kegan Paul called *Psyche Miniatures*. My notation book was published in this series, and I was sad that the diagrams and drawings, on which I had worked for months, had to be drastically reduced to fit into a miniature book.

It is of interest that it was in 1928 that Laban published his first book on *his* system of notation. I knew nothing of this at the time, and I sometimes wonder whether, if I had come across Labanotation before I had spent years evolving my own system, I would have adopted his. On balance, I doubt it, if only because I don't think that writing from the bottom of the page upward, instead of from left to right, would ever have appealed to me.

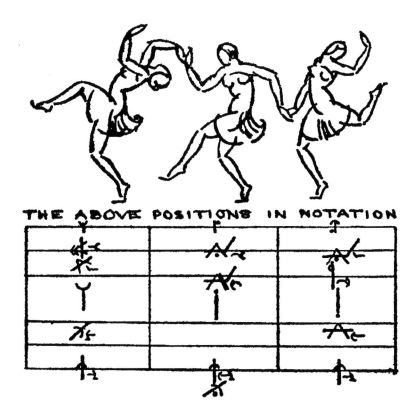

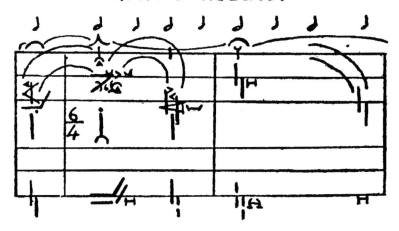

A page from Margaret Morris's *The Notation of Movement*.

Twice a week I went to St. Thomas's Hospital to take classes of physiotherapy students. Some of the Sisters also attended. I taught my basic work and improvisation, to try and give them some insight into the aesthetic approach towards remedial exercise.

For several years Sister Randell had been an enthusiastic advocate of my Movement, but when one day she called me to her room and shut the door, I wondered if perhaps the Governors had heard of my classes and disapproved of them. I was relieved to see Sister smiling warmly at me. She asked me if I had ever thought of training as a physiotherapist. It seemed that I was being criticised for treating patients, having had no medical training myself, and that *she* was being criticised for encouraging me! I replied that as I only took patients sent to me by doctors, and worked under their direction, surely that must be all right? She assured me that she herself had every confidence in me, but that the Society of Physiotherapists had pointed out that it was creating a precedent and opening the way for any unqualified person to treat patients, and that not all doctors were knowledgeable about exercises themselves.

I told Sister I had been studying anatomy and physiology on my own, and found it absorbingly interesting, so that I would be delighted to do the training, but did not see how I could possibly fit it in with my School, my theatre work, my patients and Summer Schools. She replied that if I really wanted to do it I should manage it somehow, as I had managed to do all I had done before, and that she would help me by letting me attend classes just how and when I could.

The training in those days consisted of a two-year course in massage and medical gymnastics. Electricity had just been added, but was taken afterwards, and was not obligatory as it is now. I think it took me three years instead of two, because I could hardly ever put in a whole day of classes, and often had to be absent on tour or at Summer Schools for one or two months at a time. Looking back, I wonder how I managed it at all. I had the first and second year timetables, and just went to whatever I could manage and felt I needed most, and of course

I studied on my own while away from London. But no one was more surprised than I when I took the Conjoint Examination in 1930 — and passed 'with distinction'.

I was thrilled, for it was the first and only examination I had ever done. Sister Randell was delighted, of course, and now that I was qualified I felt free to consider further developments on the remedial side of my work.

Then suddenly I was drawn back to the Dance. I received an invitation to take a group to represent Britain at a Festival of Modern Dance to be held in Florence in June 1931. It was to take place in some beautiful ornamental gardens in the city itself, with plenty of space to perform in sunlight by day, and with spot lighting in the evenings. There was to be a week of performances, planned to show what different countries were doing in developing new dance techniques. There would be no classical ballet at all. The groups could be composed of from six to fifteen dancers, and all hospitality was to be provided in Florence. I think some allowance was given towards fares, but I know it cost us quite a lot to get there.

On arrival we were met at the station by a committee of ladies, and I was presented with a bouquet. We were then escorted to our hotels, where I had a room with a private bath and a balcony overlooking the Arno and the famous Ponte Vecchio. Our hostesses would hardly leave us, and any free moment we had — and there weren't many — they rushed us off in cars to see the sights of Florence.

Unfortunately, everything had been arranged for presentation against a lovely garden setting in summer sunshine or on warm nights, but it rained continuously the whole week that we were there. It was also quite cool, though we were told this was unheard-of in Italy in June. The outdoor project had to be abandoned, and the performances transferred to the theatre, which was not very big. In some ways I preferred this, for there was a background of plain, dark curtains: but having been warned that our allotted time must allow for getting on and off the spot in the gardens where the demonstrations were to take place, this now meant that every turn had time to fill in, and we had to spend every spare minute rehearsing in the theatre, when we had expected to be free to see Florence.

I watched all the different groups with great interest. Elizabeth Duncan, Isadora's sister, was there with a group of children, for it was she who gave Isadora's troupe all the training they had. There were several schools from Germany and Austria, and representatives from the Wigman, Laban and Martha Graham schools. Our own group was very well received, and we were presented with a bronze medal, a beautiful venetian bowl and a large silver tray. We all enjoyed it tremendously. Seeing other people's creative work was most stimulating and we returned refreshed: but as usual, though we had had excellent notices in the Italian papers, our lack of a press agent meant that no news of our success reached England.

That Florentine visit made me determined to establish the Movement internationally. I had long wanted to open a school in Paris, because I loved France and wanted to spend more time there, but this was out of the question while I was training at St Thomas's. Now I began to think of France again and to realise that, as a qualified physiotherapist, it would be much easier for me to approach the French doctors and to establish the two sides of my work simultaneously. As soon as I could get away, I went over to Paris to see what could be done.

I had an introduction to a woman with a large house in the avenue de la Bourdonnais in the Invalides district. I think it was a select kind of boarding-house, but I was able to hire a big, lofty room there for classes. I also had introductions to many people likely to be interested. After I had given a demonstration, I was able to start classes at once. They soon outgrew that one large room, and I then looked for a furnished flat, where I could install a teacher, as I myself had to spend so much of my time in London. I was lucky in finding a small apartment in the boulevard Saint-Germain. It had thick carpets and rather gloomy purple velvet curtains, but it impressed our private pupils, of which we had many. A hall had still to be hired for the larger classes, however. Eventually I found a top-floor studio flat in the rue de Sèvres near the boulevard Montparnasse, and we were able to hold all our classes there.

I have an idea Mary Sykes was the first teacher I sent to Paris; and there was also a Jane Todd. I cannot remember them all, for they changed rather often, as so many wanted to go there, but of course they had to have some knowledge of French. I can't help remembering Jocelyn Gunson, whom I installed in our first flat. She was a charming and talented girl, but reputed to be hopelessly untidy. So I called one morning unexpectedly, and was delighted to find the classroom in perfect order, as she slept on the divan. I thought she had this too far forward in the room, so I pushed it back against the wall, revealing most of Jocelyn's frocks, shoes and underclothes, dirty towels, books, and papers, etc, well concealed under the divan!

Another teacher was Betsy Adlard. She was not long in Paris because she obtained a post at the International School, Geneva, where they had one of my teachers for many years, right up to the war. Betsy deserves to be mentioned because she is one of the most perfect examples of M.M.M. training, showing how it can be carried on into middle age and over. She was a lovely dancer in her youth, and now she has four grown-up sons and is a grandmother, yet she is slim and supple, runs classes near Cheltenham, and still dances beautifully.

I visited the school at Geneva once. It was fascinating to see children of so many nationalities, boys and girls, of many shades of skin, all doing M.M.M. I remember two Chinese boys were especially good at the Greek positions.

By this time, I had two teachers with me in Paris, and both were fully employed. Two students were doing half-day training — one English girl who later married the portrait painter, James Gunn, the other Irish, the daughter of the writer James Joyce, who was living in Paris at that time.

Everything went easily in Paris. The British Ambassador then was Lord Tyrrell, to whom I was fortunate enough to have an introduction from Sir Arthur and Lady Willert, whom I had met when bathing at Eden Roc. Sir Arthur had recently retired from the Foreign Office, and was an old friend of Lord Tyrrell's. I came to know Lady Willert very well; her son married one of my pupils, and when she died I missed her very much, especially in the summers at Eden Roc, where we first met.

That introduction of the Tyrrells was the most fruitful I ever had. Lord Tyrrell was a remarkable man, of small, compact stature, very determined and fearless of public opinion and stupid conventions. His daughter Ann, now the Hon. Mrs Crawshay, was hostess at the Embassy, her mother being a semi-invalid, and she, more than anyone, helped me to become established in Paris. She was especially interested in the remedial work, particularly on the maternity side, which she said would be something quite new to France; and she offered to give a reception and invite all the society women she knew, together with a few leading doctors, so that I could explain and demonstrate my ante- and post-natal exercises before this audience. I thought it was an excellent idea, but I wondered about Lord Tyrrell's reaction. She assured me that he would be delighted, and so he was.

The demonstration took place a few weeks later. In the middle of the Embassy ballroom stood an iron bedstead with a firm mattress (I wondered where it came from), with two rows of chairs in a semi-circle facing it in front; and behind it, at the far end of the room, a tea buffet was laid out. Lord Tyrrell introduced me most charmingly and it was not till I was in the middle of my talk that I noticed, as I turned back towards the bed, a row of young footmen ranged behind the buffet. They went pink with embarrassment when I explained the importance of strengthening the pelvic floor and showed the delivery exercise. But all the seats were occupied by sophisticated Parisiennes, with the doctors standing behind them, so no one seemed in the least disconcerted by the young men's presence, and it was all a great success. I acquired many private pupils as a result, some of them coming to me for breathing and relaxation to reduce tension; and others, who had recently had children, wanting their figures improved. The French doctors were interested, and arranged for me to lecture, in French, at several hospitals. Some of them also sent me patients, so I had more than enough to do.

Ann Tyrrell had heavy responsibilities, which made her tired and tense, and she slept very badly. She asked me if I would come early in the mornings before she got up, and give her lessons to help her relax: so when I was in Paris I used to arrive at the Embassy at 8.30 most mornings, and this continued for some time. I think I helped her a little, and as I liked and admired her very much we became good friends.

Ann Tyrrell introduced me to a friend who lived in Chelsea, Mrs Clifford Norton, always known as 'Peter' Norton. (She is now, in fact, Lady Norton, her husband having been Ambassador in Athens for many years.) I contacted Peter as soon as I got back to London. She was immediately interested and, having watched the work of the school, decided she would like to take lessons herself, but wanted them at her own house in Carlyle Square. As this was very near Glebe Place I agreed, and we soon became friends. She was a great skiing enthusiast, and she made up her mind that I must do a book of skiing exercises. Although I protested that I knew nothing whatever about skiing, and had no time anyway, she was persistent. She informed me that one of the best ski instructors, Hans Falkner, was coming to London shortly, so that we could work out the exercises together. As she also managed to interest a publisher in the idea, I capitulated.

Once I had started I became intensely interested. Hans Falkner showed me the movements as they should be done, and I put them into an exercise that could be practised, to music if desired. Then I did the drawings. This was not difficult: I loved drawing as much as I disliked writing, but my drawings had to be carefully checked for accuracy of the positions, as well as for the verbal descriptions, though Peter Norton was largely responsible for these.[2a]

As soon as the manuscript was delivered I went back to Paris, where the school was thriving and where I had been asked to give a course on my maternity exercises to a group of French midwives. I found that these women, who were mostly young and pretty, had much more standing in France than midwives have in England. They were expected to deal with complicated deliveries, and their importance was emphasised by the clothes they wore. In French hospitals in the 'thirties there were no nursing uniforms as we know them here. The French being essentially practical and economical, the nurses wore white overalls and aprons, with squares tied round their heads, all perfectly clean, indeed sterilised, but all rough-dried, so that there was no appearance of smartness. The overalls of the midwives were always well pressed and they wore pink squares round their heads to distinguish them from the nurses. They were very interested in my lectures, but when I showed the delivery exercise with the patient on her side — the French always place the patient flat on her back, with knees bent and legs wide apart — they appeared puzzled and amused, and a young doctor called out: '*Ah oui — ça c'est la pruderie anglaise!*'

When I next travelled to London, and I used to cross the Channel every three or four weeks — no flying in those days — I saw Sister Randell, who was delighted at the interest shown in Paris, and I think it was my idea that she and I should do a book on maternity and post-operative exercises.

For some time before we met she had been working with Dr Fairbairn on the idea of movement in relation to childbirth, and had been teaching her patients the essential movements for delivery and for strengthening the stretched muscles after the birth. My contribution was to put these movements into exercises, giving them a more carrying form, to be done in rhythmic sequence and to music where possible. I had worked these out with Sister Randell, and she had been teaching them to her students for some time past. The manuscript required some years of preparation, and it was finally published, with my illustrations, in 1936.[3] It went into two editions, and was also published in America.

In 1926 we were warned that we would have to leave the little theatre, and the Club which we had run there for fifteen years. The landlords required an entire floor for another billiard hall, although there was already one immediately below us. We then booked the Chenil Galleries, Chelsea, and various church halls for our classes until we moved to St Barnabas Hall, Pimlico. This was a large hall with a small stage, which enabled us to give some performances, and we remained there until we moved to really palatial premises, a double-fronted house at 31 Cromwell Road.

This period was fruitful in other ways. Dr Rollier, famous for discovering and proving the value of sun therapy in the treatment of surgical tuberculosis, and who had at that time about a dozen clinics under his direction at Leysin in Switzerland, watched my classes at the Chailey Homes, and told Mrs Kimmins: 'This is what I have imagined and hoped might one day be possible for my patients! Who invented this system?' Mrs Kimmins gave him my address, and he contacted me.

I was delighted to meet him and agreed to go to Leysin myself for three weeks, to work out with Dr Rollier how the exercises could be adapted to suit his various cases. It was well established that any movement of the affected part would increase inflammation. Thus, after surgical treatment complete immobilisation was prescribed, the patients being encased in plaster to ensure it. This treatment was often successful in curing the disease, but resulted in stiffening of the joints concerned. Dr Rollier considered that, though most movement must be avoided, complete immobilisation was contrary to nature, and would retard the healing process. He surrounded the affected part with sandbags, to ensure rest, while keeping it exposed to the sun for the active healing process. His theory was that, as all healing took place through the blood, to increase the rate of circulation in the rest of the body, while keeping the affected part immobilised, must increase the rate of healing in that part.

I composed a number of exercises on this basis: the breathing was suitable for all patients. My difficulty in explaining the exercises was that many of them only spoke German, though Leysin is in French Switzerland. To get the patients to expand their chests on inspiration, I learnt to say: 'Heben die

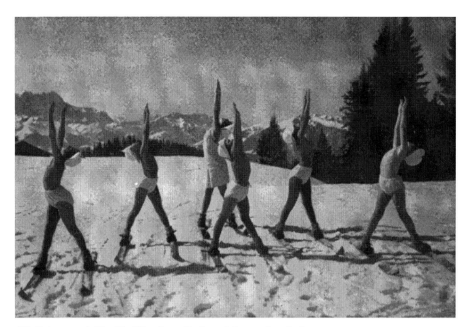

**Children at Dr Rollier's clinic at Leysin doing
corrective exercises on skis.**

Brust!' and expiration, to induce the pulling in of the abdomen, I would cry: 'Einn*zieh*-en!' That is all the German I ever learnt, and it caused great amusement to a German who tried to converse with me on the journey back, and found I could only say: '*Einnziehen! Heben die Brust!*'

The first three weeks at Leysin were unforgettable. I had never seen really deep, high-altitude snow before, and although I had no time to learn to ski or skate, I found it exhilarating. I lived with the Rolliers, but slept at a clinic opposite their house. I had a large balcony, with a bed on wheels, which I could pull outside and sleep in the open. Sometimes the snow fell on my face. I had two hot-water bottles, so that I was never cold.

The Rolliers are a remarkable family. There are four charming, intelligent daughters. They all came to my school in London at various times. Two were students and acquired the teaching diploma. For twenty years one of my teachers worked at Leysin, and Dr Rollier's daughters Madeleine and Suzanne taught at the clinics until they married.

After Dr Rollier's death everything changed. Antibiotic treatment had been discovered, and several clinics closed. Leysin has become a holiday centre, with a swimming pool and tennis courts, and skiing and skating in winter, and the clinics have been converted into hotels and *pensions*. Mme Rollier, who is in her eighties, still lives there. I spent a very happy time with her two years ago. Madeleine, who became a special friend of mine, also lives there and Suzanne, who is married to a pastor, still conducts classes.

My life in movement has certainly been varied: theatrical, remedial work as well as sport. Subsequently my activities alternated between orthopaedics, athletics and the stage. I had only recently noticed the striking similarity between the positions in my exercises and those constantly occurring in football, cricket and tennis. Tennis interested me especially, because I had seen many pictures of Suzanne Lenglen, the tennis champion.

In Paris, I demonstrated how all athletic movements were inevitably based on the opposition of one group of muscles to another, as shown and accentuated in Duncan's Greek positions. I demonstrated these and other opposition exercises, and then showed positions from photographs of Lenglen in action. She was in the audience, brought, I believe, by Ann Tyrrell.

It was already some years since Suzanne Lenglen had stopped playing; she was running a tennis school in Paris. She realised immediately that with her guidance I could compose special tennis exercises, which could be used as a basic preparatory training. She invited me to lunch at her flat in Passy, and discussed the strokes that should be incorporated into the exercises. She was a dynamic personality, stimulating to work with, and I never saw a sign of the violent temper she was reputed to possess. We evolved the exercises at her flat, where I often met other tennis stars. The only one I remember by name is Borotra, possible because his personality impressed me. He was slight, dark and like quicksilver.

As soon as the exercises were finished, Suzanne said we

must publish them; she directed me to visit Mr Evans of Heinemann's, who was a friend and admirer from her championship days. I requested an advance of £200, to be divided between us. Mr Evans was charming and eager to publish the book, but he pointed out that £200 was too much. I told him Suzanne had said that was her price, and that I was to insist, whereupon he smiled and said: 'You win — Suzanne always gets her own way!'

Before leaving Paris I had taught the exercises to one of my teachers, who worked every day at Suzanne's school. She made it compulsory for all her pupils to learn the strokes by doing our exercises before they were allowed to use a racket. They were also obliged to practice the special breathing exercises regularly. Suzanne declared that she obtained much quicker results, and the pupils had more endurance. Her tennis-star friends were impressed by this and several of them insisted on coming to me for private lessons, to develop their breathing and improve their style.

The book[4] went into two editions and was later published in France. But if it is ever reprinted, I shall have to do new drawings, as I depicted a male figure in long, flapping trousers.

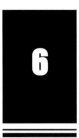

SOMEONE ELSE WHO WAS A TREMENDOUS HELP to the Movement was a curious, to me rather mysterious, man named Howard Evans. When I met him he was Headmaster of Betteshanger Preparatory School for Boys, and I was introduced to him through Lord Cholmondeley, whose two sons attended the school. He and Lady Cholmondeley had been present at the Charity Matinée I gave at the Savoy Theatre for the Chailey Homes. I had explained my method, which was demonstrated by pupils from my school as well as by the disabled children themselves, and Lord Cholmondeley was so much impressed that he wrote at once to Howard Evans, suggesting that he should contact me and try to engage one of my teachers for Betteshanger, which he did. I was of course delighted to fall in with the idea. At first I sent a male instructor, but once the work was well established, and a resident teacher was required, one of my girls took over and proved satisfactory.

Howard Evans was an extraordinary person. He was quite small and not particularly good-looking, but he had great charm of manner and a keen sense of humour; he was always good company and a delightful host. At the school he was inclined to be domineering and dictatorial, but he got results! How he came to be Headmaster of Betteshanger and how long he had been there I never learnt: but he told me that previously he had been a dress designer in New York, so that he knew about the rag trade, as well as advertising, to which he turned later. Altogether a strange background for a Headmaster, but to judge by results it was a good one. He was extremely popular with the parents, for whom he ran a kind of house party in his own wing of the

My Life in Movement

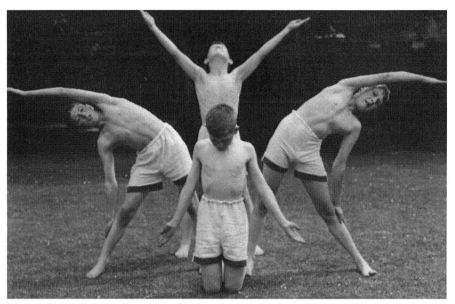

Boys from Betteshanger School.

schoolhouse every weekend, and these gatherings offered all
the attractions of a luxurious Country Club. A different selection
of parents was invited each week, and there was excellent food
and a profusion of drinks before and during dinner, with card
games afterwards. I myself was often invited and met many
leading doctors, army men, civil servants and their wives. All of
them praised Howard and were delighted to visit their children at
school.

Howard did a great deal to establish my Movement as a
basic physical training for men and boys. His personal interest
in the Movement made the Betteshanger boys take it seriously.
Howard used to arrange impressive end-of-term demonstrations, for which he would rehearse them repeatedly until they
achieved a good team effect. At one of these demonstrations
that I attended, an old army colonel standing beside me
complimented me: but later I saw him looking worried, and he
asked me: 'Do you teach girls too?' I naturally replied that most
of my work was with girls, whereupon he said: 'Oh, I shouldn't
like this for *girls*!', and walked away. I was delighted; I was so
tired of being told it was very good for girls, but not strenuous

enough for boys!

In these Betteshanger demonstrations we had, of course, emphasised the breathing exercises, and the basic preparation for athletics and games. Later on Howard took a team of boys on a tour of schools in America, demonstrating M.M.M., and they were widely publicised. Howard had great aesthetic sensibility, and he was an admirer of my own dancing. He regretted that I danced so little and he was always finding me new records, Bach, Brahms, Rimsky-Korsakov, Stravinsky. He was very musical and I was invariably inspired by the records he found for me. When I said I had no time to compose more dances, he insisted I visit Betteshanger, where he shut me into a room with a gramophone and told me to get on with it! I did, and composed some of my best dances. It is still a mystery to me how Howard induced people to do whatever he wished.

Some years later, quite suddenly, like our good agent Briggs, Howard died. I never found out the cause; he was only in his forties. I missed him as a friend and as an impresario. Of all the people who have believed in my Movement and helped me, Howard was the most interested in me as a dancer. He bullied me into composing new dances and never lost an opportunity of stating that my Movement was great because I was a great dancer.

Peter Norton was more interested in the Movement as a whole, with its wide range of possibilities. She felt I had found and unified the essentials in movement for establishing and maintaining health in human beings of any age, and for preparatory training in sports and athletics. She recognised that the combination of the aesthetic and medical aspects was only possible because I approached the question of physical education as an artist. She fully appreciated the educational value of the aesthetic side of my Movement: but although she saw many of our shows and admired some of the dances, I don't think she ever believed — as I still believe — that the method was capable of producing great dancers for the theatre.

On the educational, athletic and remedial sides, however, Peter Norton had total affinity with me. She was indignant that my work was not more widely known and officially recognised in order that a training college for teachers could have been established, and children in all schools, including those for the disabled, would have benefited. We were already sending visiting teachers to several private schools, but in spite of my efforts I failed completely to obtain official recognition. Over the years I gave many demonstrations which were always enthusiastically received and often attended by directors of education: but when I had interviews with them, asking them to try out my method by making a controlled test for six months at a state school, with half the school continuing on the old P.T. method, and half being put on to mine, all the children to be medically examined before and after the test, I always received the same answer: the matter would have to be referred to the Ling Association (at that time the controlling P.T. organisation), and each time they refused, reminding the director that unauthorised teachers could not take classes in a state school. They had accepted the Swedish system and they would not admit that it could possibly be improved upon. It was certainly better than the old army drill, but still far too tense, and all the movements were done to words of command.

The directors of education themselves seemed to be helpless. The last one I saw was Sir Charles Trevelyan, a charming, cultured man, who was, I think, sincerely interested in what I showed him and really sorry to be so powerless; but anything relating to physical training had to be referred to 'the experts'. He suggested that I should give demonstrations at physical training colleges. I wasted much time and money in fares, giving demonstrations, which the colleges were pleased to have as entertainment for their students, and the Headteachers made speeches of thanks; but they always pointed out to me afterwards that any free kind of movement and improvisation would be quite impossible for large local authority school classes.

At that time the regulation gym tunic was still dark-blue serge, and worn with black stockings, and a long-sleeved, white, well-starched blouse. I remember watching a demonstration at the Dartford Physical Training College (Madame Osterberg's). Every time the arms came sharply to the sides there was a loud crackling of starched sleeves.

I called on Miss Wilkie, then Head of the Chelsea College of Physical Education, and induced her to visit my school to see a demonstration. She was politely appreciative, saying it was a beautiful spectacle, but that she felt it belonged to the theatre. She could find no connection between aesthetic movement and gymnastics, and she did not approve of our tunics, saying they exposed too much of the body.

Soon afterwards, Miss Wilkie invited me to her college, to see a class at work. I sat beside her on the platform and watched an almost exact reproduction of the class I had seen at Dartford with the same crackle of starched sleeves; I was able to admire the precision of movement and the balance and agility of apparatus work, although I have never been able to see what relation apparatus work bears to the life and movement of the ordinary human being: I suggested that freer and more flowing movements might be added, giving some opportunity for freedom of expression. Miss Wilkie would not hear of this as it would interfere with accuracy and precision. I then suggested some softer kind of tunic, pointing out that the heavy serge pleats undeniably hid faults of posture, and that the black stockings should be discarded. She was horrified and said that the uniform would never be changed.

These two discouraging contacts convinced me that it was useless to attempt to interest the P.T. colleges. It seems to me that the British authorities are unwilling to accept any innovations or improvements if these come from one of themselves, but that they are always ready to spend money on sending people abroad to investigate, and often to adopt, new foreign methods. For example, the Ling method of gymnastics that was introduced from Sweden, and, more recently, the Laban method of free dance from Germany, which has been officially recognised and is now taught in state schools.

Peter Norton, however, was not to be discouraged. She said we must get a better headquarters for the school. If we had an important building where we could establish a proper training college, we would, given really good publicity, be bound to gain recognition. We therefore formed a non-profit-making company, appealing to all parents and friends for support, which many of them gave: and the search for suitable premises began.

In 1935 we found a large, double-fronted house at 31 Cromwell Road, facing the Natural History Museum. It had thirty rooms and two staircases: a steep and narrow one out of sight at the back of the house; and a beautiful well staircase spiralling up from the front hall. This, when I first saw it, was painted in black and gold, which I at once changed to white. The rooms were large and lofty, including a ballroom with five windows across the front of the house, which made a big classroom. On this floor there were wide balconies overlooking a fair-sized garden, a square lawn backed by big trees. The back of this garden adjoined that of the French Lycée, where we held classes later on, our teachers making their way there over the garden wall.

Peter Norton had been in publicity before her marriage, so she was invaluable and had many influential friends. Ann Tyrrell, by that time the Hon. Mrs Crawshay, consented to preside at the opening. There was a demonstration in the garden, and refreshments were served. The house looked beautiful. We had spent as much as we could afford on redecoration, and had bought second-hand furniture, which the students painted in clear, bright colours. This time our publicity was excellent, and we soon had a big influx of students.

For a long time I had wanted to establish my Movement in Scotland for which, ever since I had visited it on tour with theatrical companies as a child, I had always felt an extraordinary affinity. Whenever we went to Glasgow in those early touring days, my first thought had been to get to Loch Long, walking up the side of the loch from Whistlefield to Arrochar, where I would take a train back in time for the evening performance. Often it rained, and I would return soaked. At first my mother came with me on these expeditions, for she also loved them. In later years a friend in the company would be my companion. As soon as we reached Edinburgh I could not wait to climb to the top of Arthur's Seat. My mother always used to climb with me to the very top: but later on it was harder to find a companion for this fairly stiff climb, and I often had to go alone.

Later still, of course, my friendship with J.D. Fergusson, and his active interest and cooperation in my Movement, became the determining factor in my decision to start branch schools up there. I decided that Edinburgh, as the first city, must be my starting point, and I travelled there with Betty Simpson, who had taken over from me the Chailey Homes and Dr Rollier's Clinics at Leysin. She had also spent a year in America in 1932 as resident M.M. teacher at the very modern Halcyon Farm School.

On our arrival in Edinburgh in 1935, Betty and I stayed at the Caledonia Hotel, feeling that we must begin our search for premises as near the centre as possible: and almost at once we were lucky enough to find an upper flat in South Charlotte Street, just off the West End of Princes Street, an ideal position. The house was an old one, with large rooms and a charming staircase, winding up to the top floor. We took it at once, and arranged for complete interior redecoration in light, clear colours. The classrooms were always pale, eau-de-nil green, as this was most becoming to the skin, and bare arms and legs were *de rigueur*. Other rooms were pale pink or white. Meanwhile we attended furniture sales and collected an extraordinary amount of junk, dozens of chairs (mostly deficient), large and small tables etc. Later these were all painted — as had been done prior to the opening in London — in the approved M.M. colours, and many people remarked on the attractive final effect. In these days of 'do-it-yourself' decorations this may not seem a very original way of treating large empty premises, but at that time it was an innovation.

From the start, the Edinburgh school was an unqualified success. It always paid its way, largely due to a most efficient principal, Gwen Barham, one of my best teachers, and because, as a result of its excellent central situation, we soon had more private pupils (for reducing, correcting flat feet etc), than we could accept. These came to us, as well as a satisfactory number of dancing pupils, following our public demonstrations, when students were enrolled.

We were lucky in the City's Director of Education, Mr J. B. Frizell, who was an exceptional person. He was always accessible and encouraging, and was so impressed by my demonstration of exercises and aesthetic work for the physically disabled that he arranged for groups to be sent to us by ambulance twice a week. It is one of my greatest regrets that when the 1939 war started, we had to close the Edinburgh School. I find it hard to forgive Gwen Barham, who insisted on joining up. The school could have continued, and might indeed have done valuable therapeutic work during the war years.

The Glasgow School opened in 1936. Again I was lucky in finding a flat in a central position, 299 West George Street, at the corner of Blythswood Square: but this school was less successful. Wealthy people mostly live outside Glasgow, so we never had the same steady flow of private pupils and children's classes as in Edinburgh. Here too the Director of Education, Dr Stewart Mackintosh, always appreciated what we were trying to do, and was as helpful as he could be, but there was a lack of cooperation. He wished to start experimental classes in the schools, but he was always blocked by the teachers, or by the Physiotherapist Society.

Dr Mackintosh introduced me to the Matron of the East Park Home for the Disabled, a charming and intelligent woman, who was anxious to have the services of one of my teachers: but in order to get classes started there I had to offer one without fee. The Matron told me that if she applied to the authorities for money to pay a teacher, she would most certainly be refused, whereas if we could show at a demonstration what the disabled children could be made to do, and how much they enjoyed it, she hoped officialdom would be convinced that it was worth doing.

A year later a demonstration was given at the Kelvinside Special School. We had a perfect day and were able to give it out of doors. The children were wonderful, and their obvious enjoyment was so infectious that no one could help being impressed. Afterwards congratulatory speeches were made by Dr Macintosh and Mr Kennedy Fraser, who was in charge of 'Scottish Schools for the Handicapped', and said that what I had to offer must be used, and to judge from the enthusiastic applause everyone agreed. The Matron of the East Park Home was delighted, and so was I. At last, I thought — not for the first time — something was going to happen. But nothing ever did. We carried on with the classes until the Matron retired. Then they stopped, for the new Matron disapproved.

This was one of my biggest disappointments. I had hoped I would be asked to give special courses for teachers working with disabled children, or to train students who wanted to specialise in this work. When I talked with Dr Mackintosh and Mr Kennedy Fraser (a son of Mrs Kennedy Fraser, famous for collecting and publishing *Songs of the Hebrides*), they both said they could only engage teachers from the recognised training colleges. When I approached these colleges, the result was exactly the same as in England. They were delighted to have a demonstration, as they told me they liked their students to see other methods. But they never wanted to make such methods or ideas the subject of any serious study. The result has been, of course, a process of gradual change, serge tunics and black stockings being replaced by coloured tunics and free movement and improvisation: but it has come about without the basic knowledge of design in movement which I could have provided, and which is essential to give variety and maintain interest over a long period.

In 1935 the School of Physiotherapy at the Royal Infirmary, Glasgow, having already heard of Sister Randell's maternity work at St Thomas's Hospital, and of the exercises I had devised under her guidance, learnt also that I had started a branch in Edinburgh. They asked if one of our teachers could visit Glasgow twice a week and teach their students at the Western Infirmary. This we did for a year until the Glasgow School was opened in 1936. After that, their students came to us two mornings a week and at the end of their training took our Maternity Exercise Diploma, because at that time the physiotherapy training did not include maternity work. This continued for fifteen years, by which time training for maternity work had been included in the physiotherapy training.

It is amazing how often I have come across physiotherapists who trained at that time, and all of them have told me how much they enjoyed and benefited by the classes at the M.M.M. School, and that whenever possible they use our exercises in preference to any others. Many friends who have come across them quite independently as patients have reported the same thing. I still hope that one day, although I don't expect to live to see it, all physiotherapists may benefit by what I believe I have to give them: namely a fundamental knowledge of form and design, and the ability to approach the problems of corrective exercise with the vision of an artist.

7

MEANWHILE THE LONDON SCHOOL in its new Cromwell Road premises was a hive of activity. Dorothy Gates was principal, an excellent and most reliable teacher. Her husband, Eric Gates, was an international soccer player. He smiled when I said my exercises were just as suitable for men as for women, until one day his wife persuaded him to try our Greek opposition-positions, and kept him at it for an hour. The next day he could hardly move! This convinced him that the exercises were tough enough even for footballers, and he found that they supplied the best possible out-of-season training, which he himself practised regularly during the summer months. This, and Lord Cholmondeley's interest, turned my mind more and more to the application of my work as a preparatory training for all sports and athletics.

Since getting classes started at Betteshanger School, Lord Cholmondeley himself had been taking regular private lessons, and it was his conviction that mine was the best physical training system that had yet been evolved, and his insistence that I must write a book about it, that eventually made me produce *Basic Physical Training*.[5] This became the elementary text-book for all our students, as the fundamental exercises are the same for both sexes, but I illustrated the exercises with masculine-looking figures, and included a few from higher standards to give stronger knee-bending work and to develop spring.

This book has been out of print for over twenty-five years. I told Heinemann it was a required text-book for all our students, which would have ensured permanent steady sales, but it was found necessary to break down the blocks during the war owing to shortage of material and the post-war expense of new blocks has prevented its re-issue. All the libraries had copies originally, but our students used to take them out and fail to return them, saying they were lost and paying the necessary fine; so I doubt if the book is to be found in any library today.

Dr Jack Lovelock, the Olympic runner, was one of our most enthusiastic supporters. His medical training enabled him to appreciate the anatomical and physiological structure of the exercise: and he said the Greek positions, which he learned to do beautifully himself, should be included in the daily training of all runners, being an exaggeration of the movements used in running. He also believed that our free running, with long springing steps and free relaxed swinging of the arms, should be practised by all runners as a preparatory training. Obviously, it is not possible to run that way on the track; but Lovelock believed

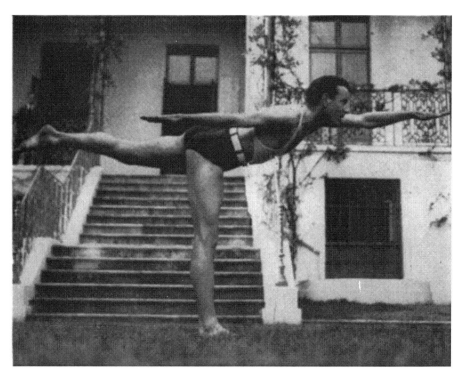

Roland Harper, Olympic hurdler, demonstrating at the London Training School, 1937.

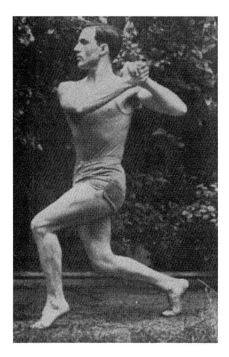

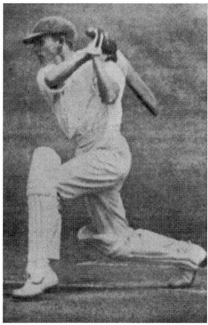

Illustrations from the prospectus of the Basic Physical Training Association, 1938. (Below) Donald Bradman.

that the relaxed stretching of the muscles would tend to reduce tension and fatigue on the track as well. It was a great loss to my Movement when he died some years ago.

Another distinguished athlete who believed in our exercises was Roland Harper (Olympic hurdler, 1932), now Director of Physical Education, University of Manchester. Again it was the opposition of the Greek positions and the balance that appealed to him particularly, and he suggested that we alter the arms in one special balance to make it approximate that of a hurdler. I did so, and to this day it remains 'the Hurdler's Balance'.

That summer Suzanne Lenglen came to London for the Tennis at Wimbledon. One day she took me with her, and introduced me to 'Bunny' Austin, the great star of the moment, who was not playing that day. Suzanne told him how she used my work in her school, and of how pleased she was with the results, and he was at once interested. He said lack of staying power always kept him back, that he felt his breathing was to blame for this, and asked if I would take him on as a pupil. I was delighted, and he had lessons from me for about a year, saying they helped him a lot, and that if only he had known of me when he started playing tennis, his stamina would have been doubled, and I believe it would.

While she was in London, Suzanne was invited by Lady Crosfield, one of the leading tennis hostesses of the 'thirties, to a big tennis party she was giving, and to demonstrate her teaching methods to the guests. Suzanne telephoned me, saying this would be a good opportunity to interest people in my tennis exercises, and that I must come and demonstrate for her. I was quite happy to show my own exercises, but when Suzanne said I must also show the correct way to hold the racket etc, while she only gave verbal explanations, I felt inadequate. But when the time came, I had been well coached by Suzanne.

The party was held at a large house with extensive grounds and several tennis courts, where the guests were to play tennis after our demonstration: and when Suzanne had finished her talk, and I had shown my exercises, we were overwhelmed with congratulations. People crowded round me saying how beautiful

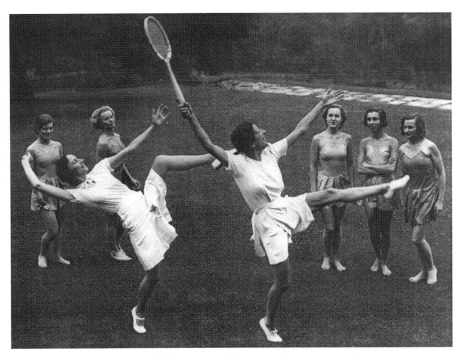

Suzanne Lenglen and Margaret Morris demonstrating a tennis exercise.

the exercises were, and how perfectly I had demonstrated the strokes, and then added, to my embarrassment: 'Now, of course, we are just longing to see you play!' When I replied: 'But I *don't!*' everyone gasped. I have never seen so much astonishment and disbelief registered on so many faces, and I was obliged to give a detailed account of my theatrical, aesthetic, and later medical background to explain how I had trained athletes as well as dancers, but had never had time to play any games myself.

Everyone seemed greatly interested, and I am sure I could have enrolled many pupils for tennis exercises if I had had time to follow up the demonstration: but as always throughout my life, too many things seemed to be happening all at once. I was planning the opening of a school in Manchester, Lord Cholmondeley had made contacts for me on the athletic side, and meanwhile, my professional dancing students were clamouring for more attention to the theatrical side of my work.

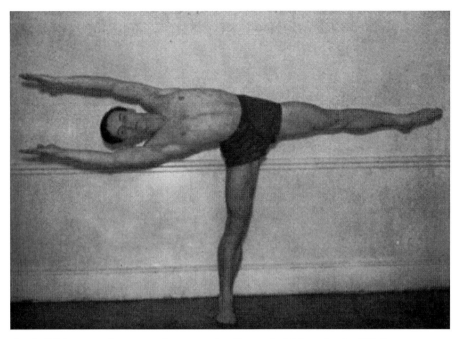

Jack Skinner, dancer, demonstrating at Aldershot, 1935.

About this time a body called the British Army manifested a sudden desire to know about my Movement. I had a letter from Colonel Wand-Tetley, then in charge of the Army Training School at Aldershot, saying that the medical and P.T. staff would be interested to see a demonstration of my methods. I was naturally pleased and we planned a striking demonstration to be led by our principal dancer, Jack Skinner, with five of our male students. This was well rehearsed, and on the appointed day a party of seven, of whom I was the only female, went down to Aldershot. An army car met us, Colonel Wand-Tetley welcomed us, and we gave our demonstration, which I conducted as usual with an explanatory talk, in one of the big gymnasia.

As always, I found the doctors the most receptive. They could appreciate the logic of my arguments regarding the anatomical and physiological aspects of the exercises, and they seemed to understand the importance of breathing and the opposition muscle work of the Greek positions. One doctor told me he was particularly impressed by what I said about foot exercise, because keeping the feet in condition is always a major problem in the army. I stressed the value of exercising part of each day with bare feet, to use the small intrinsic muscles, which do not function properly if shoes are worn, even soft ones: and I was assured that a daily routine of exercises with bare feet would be started without delay.

We were then asked to demonstrate a few of the simpler exercises a second time, so that the P.T. staff could include them in their classes, and Colonel Wand-Tetley asked me if I would return in six weeks' time to see if they were being taught correctly. I agreed at once to do so.

When I arrived, it was quite impressive. I saw a large class in shorts and bare feet doing my exercises. The instructors had done quite a good job, but I had to correct one of the floor exercises, pelvic turning. In this exercise, the arms and shoulders are kept on the ground, while one leg is taken across to give the pelvic turning movement. The class were lifting the leg and *dropping* it across, using mainly the recti muscles, whereas the leg should be taken across near the ground, thus using the oblique muscles. The doctors at once realised that the mistake reduced the value of the exercise and promised that it would be corrected. I was also asked to write two articles for the *Army Journal of Physical Training*: it seemed that my theories were being taken seriously at last.

I sensed, however, that the P.T. instructors were not too pleased with my innovations. Being in the army, they had to obey orders, but I wondered how long it would be before they managed to side-track them. Jack Skinner had given a brilliant display, well supported by our students. He had wonderful control of balance, and great elevation, doing spectacular leaps, and the army instructors had the grace to congratulate him.

As Jack is the best male dancer we ever produced, I want to say something about him here. He came to me in the early Chelsea days, a very shy little boy of eight. Although he was always a good pupil, he was thin, and slow to develop the latent talents he evidently possessed; and no one would ever have guessed that one day he would be the star dancer in *Oklahoma*, and would now be touring the world with his wife Joy, in a highly paid dance act called 'Emerson and Jayne'. He became our principal dancer in the 'twenties, having passed my ten standards of exercises. He was a splendid teacher and dance producer, always entirely reliable and devoted to his art, and never sparing himself, or others, at rehearsals.

I think Colonel Wand-Tetley was genuinely impressed by Jack's display. He said he would like to try some of the exercises himself, and asked if he could bring two or three of his officers to 31 Cromwell Road, and if I would give them a few lessons personally. At the same time he asked me to be careful that the press did not hear of it. Of course I had to agree to this, but it was disappointing, as I could have obtained valuable publicity from an announcement that the British Army were using my exercises.

In the same way, I had also achieved notable results in my medical work, but if I had made them known I should have been accused of professional advertising: so the Movement as a whole never benefited.

Meanwhile, I invited Colonel Wand-Tetley and his officers to be my guests. I gave them, I think, four lessons, and afterwards entertained them to a health lunch of salad and fruit, which they seemed to enjoy, though I daresay they got a steak on their way back to Aldershot. I enjoyed those sessions. The officers asked intelligent questions, and seemed to appreciate the value of what I taught them. One of them, a good-looking dark young man, confided to me that his wife was expecting a baby. He had heard I taught maternity exercises, and begged me to show him a few, so that he could help his wife. This was of course most irregular, for as a physiotherapist I was pledged to treat patients only on the authority of a doctor or surgeon: but I argued to myself that if I taught the young man I was *not* treating a patient, and I could not but admire his complete lack of embarrassment and genuine anxiety to learn. He lay on the floor and learned the 'delivery exercise', with its special breathing, and then the 'pelvic floor tensing' to avoid prolapse after delivery. I was careful not to show him anything that might be dangerous if not properly taught; but as I am still a physiotherapist and a member of the obstetric section, I hope if they read this I won't be thrown out!

During 1937, Lord Cholmondeley asked us to give a demonstration in the grounds of his beautiful home, Houghton Hall in Norfolk. We had been sending a teacher for some time to hold classes locally, and the demonstration was well attended and impressive. The park is lovely, with white peacocks, which made a profound impression on me. Lord and Lady Cholmondeley were wonderful hosts, I stayed the night, but could hardly sleep for my admiration of the beautiful four-poster bed with rich brocade curtains.

Lord Cholmondeley was delighted at the experimental classes at Aldershot and at Colonel Wand-Tetley's coming to me for lessons with some of his officers. He felt now was the time to start a men's training college. I never liked this idea, as I have always believed in co-education, separation of the sexes being in my view entirely unnatural, and the cause of much psychological disturbance in later life.

However, I appreciated that the fact of my being a female, as well as a dancer, made it difficult to launch anything with army P.T. or the training of athletes under my name. So in 1938 the Basic Physical Training Association was formed under the chairmanship of Lord Cholmondeley, and a council of management of thirty- two.

As a result it was arranged to start a school of Basic Physical Training at Loughborough College. Captain A.M. Webster was the Head; one of my male teachers was instructor of B.P.T. with coaches for athletics, games etc, but this school also became a war casualty. (*Illustration from B.P.T. prospectus on page 84.*)

In 1938 I started the branch in Manchester, sending Isabel Jeayes to organise, with a young teacher to take the classes. She made a wonderful job of it, finding and taking a flat, seeing to the furnishing and redecoration — all as usual painted in the M.M. colours — and organising advance publicity, at which she was excellent. I went up for the opening demonstration, and found Isabel had arranged interviews for me with the Health and Education Authorities and a series of talks at the leading stores.

These all led to requests for classes, and the school started remarkably well.

Isabel actually came into my life through the Stonefield Maternity Home, Blackheath, where her children, Ruth and David had been born, and where all the patients did my Maternity Exercises. Dr Pink, knowing Isabel's interest in dancing, asked her to meet me; he told me she had been brilliant in her youth at gymnastics and games. She had done Natural Movement with Margaret Einert of Liverpool, who had trained with Ruth St Denis, and had also attended one of my Summer Schools at Antibes.

Isabel was a qualified teacher before her marriage, but longed to do more dancing; she came first to evening classes, then attended Intensive Courses, taking three of my Diplomas, and joining the staff at 31 Cromwell Road, but she proved herself useful in so many other ways, helping me draft letters, describing my exercises in words for my books, doing publicity for shows, and even making my complicated dance costumes, that it was not until she went to Manchester that she was able to use her talents for organisation and making contacts. Unfortunately this school, which started so well, became another war casualty.

That same year we opened a branch in Aberdeen, directed by Martha Grant (now married to James Arnott, Head of the Drama Department of the University of Glasgow). This too made an excellent start, and soon there was more work than the teachers could cope with. We were especially lucky in that Professor Baird, now Sir Dugald Baird, who was then Professor of Gynaecology at the Forester Hill Hospital, was really interested in our maternity work, and at once engaged a teacher to work at his hospital daily.

Once again it was the war that brought this school to an end so soon after its start. Martha now says she deeply regrets that she closed it up, for whatever happens women go on producing babies and it could certainly have continued: but it is easy to be wise after the event. She fully appreciated the privilege of working in such close co-operation with Professor Baird as I did, and was very sad when the association came to an end. I had hoped some day to find time to work with Professor Baird myself, and to gain more first hand experience on the delivery side. Since that time much progress has been made in ante-natal and actual delivery work: but I feel the importance of teaching really efficient post-natal exercises — for circulation, quick recovery, and to prevent prolapse — during the time the patients are in hospital, is still not fully realised. Very little is done on this side, partly because the physiotherapists are always overworked, and a few minutes' personal attention to each patient is essential.

In Aberdeen my work alternated as usual between the remedial and theatrical sides: but the theatre had been my first love and even now when I go backstage I feel like a homing pigeon. When I returned to London I plunged straight into a theatrical project. At this time, I had many good dancers, including several men. Jack Skinner, who had done so well in the Aldershot demonstrations, was determined on a theatrical career, and I had one outstandingly good girl, Audrey Seed, who later joined the Ballet Jooss, and there met her husband, a musician: so we planned for a small group of four men and six girls.

For hours we discussed what the group should be called. My own name was by then better known in medical than in theatrical circles, so I felt that this time it would be as well to use a different name altogether. Eventually we concocted one from two Eastern words meaning light and strength, and decided on the 'Ashnur Dancers', and the name was registered in 1936. This sounded oriental and I hoped would prove intriguing, and as I had been influenced by Eastern art in creating my Movement it was justified. We prepared a programme of short ballets and dances, opening with an exercise sequence to music specially composed by Hugh Bradford, our pianist for many years. For this I designed new tunics, a brassiere and short kilted skirts for the girls, and just bathing trunks for the men, all in jade green. This item made an excellent opening, and was always very well received.

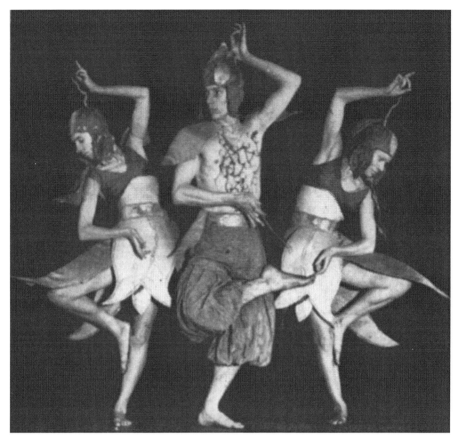

**Jack Skinner (above) and Elizabeth Cameron (opposite)
in dances they composed, at the Fortune Theatre, 1937.**

To launch the new venture I took the little Fortune Theatre by Drury Lane for a week, and it was quite successful: but our notices were not spectacular enough to make the big public rush to see the Ashnur Dancers. In spite of this I think the troupe would have got sufficient bookings, if not in England certainly abroad, had not the rumours of war already started.

In April 1937, I was asked to present the Ashnur Dancers on TV. This was our second TV show, the first being in October 1936, when we produced a half-hour programme of dances introduced by Miss Jasmine Bligh. I think I am right in saying that this was only the second dance show on television, the Ballet Rambert being the first, two weeks previously. In 1937 we

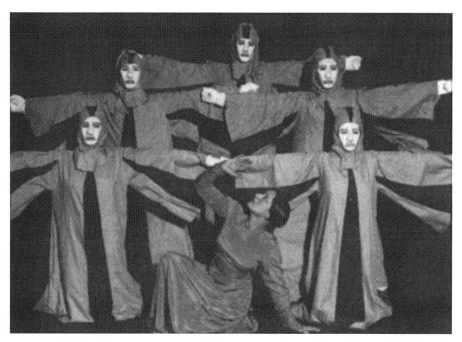

presented three more TV programmes, the first two demonstrating M.M.M. exercises and improvisation, and the last, the skiing exercises I had created with Hans Falkner, director of an Austrian ski school, who came over to demonstrate them.

The end of 1938 saw me back again in Paris, but I was already too late for the Ashnur Dancers: no one wanted to book foreign acts at a time of international crisis. Yet the Paris School was flourishing and the Cannes branch, run by Avril Gilmore and Kitty Clark, who later taught in New York, was also doing well.

I took up my remedial work again in Paris, and had many patients sent to me by one of the leading women doctors, Dr Eliet, a most charming and cultured woman. Passing through Paris only two years ago, I was delighted to find she was still in practice and I went to see her; she urged me to return to work in Paris and said she would send me many patients. In the spring of 1939, Ann Tyrrell resumed her lessons with me, and got me interested in doing a book on golf exercises, for she was an enthusiastic golfer. She introduced me to the Pro at her golf club, a man called Boomer, who liked the idea, so I started working with him. He showed me all the strokes and the way they should be done, and I composed an exercise for each one that could be repeated, with or without music, in a rhythmic pattern. Boomer argued that in golf, more than in any other game, anxiety inhibited many good players from doing their best. In practising an exercise, particularly to music, there is no anxiety, and the correct way of making a stroke is put, by constant repetition, into the subconscious. In time, it therefore becomes easier to do a stroke the right way than the wrong way. This simple, logical theory was never fully formulated in relation to golf. When I returned to England, although I taught the golf exercises with marked success to several pupils, I lost contact with Boomer and the book was never written, because of the outbreak of the Second World War.

At this time one of the teachers at the Paris School was a young Russian girl called Rita. She had been educated in France, and she carried on after the other teachers had returned to England. When finally the School had to be closed, she left Paris, taking with her only a suitcase and the gramophone with the M.M.M. records. Through a friend, she obtained a post in a convent high up in the Massif Central in France, where she taught my Movement to the children in the convent, and English to young priests at a near-by seminary, for the duration of the war. Then she married a French judge, Daniel Prost, had four children, and now, in 1969, she is teaching M.M.M. in Nouméa, New Caledonia, in the French South Pacific.

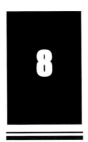

8

IN 1939 WHEN WAR WAS DECLARED I was spending the summer as usual with friends near the Château des Enfants, now La Résidence du Cap on the Cap d'Antibes. As it was their home, they meant to stay there as long as possible. I waited till the stampede of the English to get home was over, and then had a long but uneventful journey in an almost empty train. It took two whole days to reach Paris, but as I had a large hamper of food with me, it wasn't too bad.

Back in London I found that all that I had worked for during more than thirty years was crumbling to pieces around me. At the outbreak of war I had seven schools in Europe: London, Manchester, Edinburgh, Glasgow, Aberdeen, Paris and Cannes. The British schools outside London could have been kept going if I had had the staff to run them: but most of my girls got war fever, and the men were called up. I could derive no comfort from feelings of patriotism, because to me all wars were utterly and entirely wrong, and I could not believe that good could ever come out of evil. As a child, I had been told what dreadful wars there had been in the past, and how cruel and savage people used to be, but I was assured that, now we were more civilised, these things could no longer happen. But here we were in the midst of the Second World War, with far worse horrors than ever before, because more calculated and on a far bigger scale. I became completely disillusioned, and was thankful I was not a man, for I knew that I would be incapable of killing anyone, even in self-defence. As for pulling a lever to drop a bomb, that seemed to me even worse, in that it meant killing mostly quite innocent people.

I was very pleased when one of my H.Q. teachers, Claire Cassidy, already experienced in training students for diplomas, obtained a post at Pendragon School, Reading. The Headmaster, Dennis March, became enthusiastic over our work, and an M.M.M. Teachers' Training Centre was started there. Later a school theatre was built and many interesting shows produced by Claire Cassidy.

In 1939, Fergusson came to London but would not stay there. He had spent one war in England and said he would spend the next in Scotland. All good Scots as they grow older seem to be drawn back, like the salmon, to their own country. He did not want to return to Edinburgh: he had been educated there, but had left it in 1905 to settle in Paris, because the art life of Edinburgh was completely sterile, with its refusal to recognise any modern movement. The painters of the Glasgow School were called 'the Wild Men of the West', and the Scottish Academy rejected even Peploe. Fergusson's family were from Perthshire, and he wanted to go to Glasgow as the main Highland city, and try to help the young painters there. So I decided that, as I could only keep one school going, it would have to be Glasgow.

I therefore took up my quarters at the Glasgow School, where Betty Simpson, Jan Wills and Anne Cornock-Taylor were already working, believing, as I did, that it was more important to carry on with the skilled work they were doing, and had been trained for, than to rush into unskilled war work that could be done, and better done, by countless others.

I was nearly fifty: but I was full of enthusiasm, and thrilled to be living at last in Scotland, which I had loved for so long, and I was determined to make a success of that school. The Scots were fundamentally a dancing nation, so I decided to start with an amateur group and to form a club, as I had done in London during the First World War. Out of this, if we could get enough students training for the theatre, a professional company might emerge. History was repeating itself, but I refused to be discouraged. I would start all over again, with thirty years of experience behind me.

I have already described the lack of cafés and informal artistic meeting places in London at the time of the First World War. And in Glasgow in 1939 it was even worse. The people of Glasgow are warm and hospitable, and it was easier to get invited to their homes than it was to those of the Londoners. But the atmosphere of a private house, however friendly and interested, cannot provide the stimulus and freedom of inns or cafés open to the public, where writers, painters and students congregate. Lacking these, a club seemed an absolute necessity.

That being agreed, there arose the question of a name. This time I did not want to use my own, Fergusson had taught me how independent the Scots were, and I did not want them to feel I was trying to impose something on them from outside. My idea was to help create a club and a company to be run for Scots by Scots. I could lay no claim to Scottish blood myself, but I was certainly Celtic, bring Irish on one side and Welsh on the other; so I suggested the Celtic Ballet Club, the word ballet to suggest the theatre company that I hoped would eventually evolve from it.

Having decided my general policy on these lines, I wrote to Sir Patrick Dolan, the Lord Provost of Glasgow, requesting an interview, which he at once granted. I found him a charming and intelligent Irishman, and we got on very well, because he was at once interested in all I had to suggest. He recognised the real need for a cultural club in Glasgow, there being till then only one, the old Art Club, which was for men only. Moreover it had a big annual subscription, which no struggling artist could afford. I told Sir Patrick I wanted to organise a public meeting to advertise the venture. He promptly offered to chair the meeting.

Accordingly I hired a hall at Glasgow's Commercial College in Pitt Street, sent out circulars and contacted all the papers. Attendance was surprisingly good. Sir Patrick introduced me and the plan in general terms, and I then spoke of my ambition to form a Celtic Ballet, explaining that I proposed to start it as an amateur organisation, holding evening classes twice a week with the object, when we were ready, of giving performances in aid of war charities. I asked those interested in this scheme to enrol as members of the Celtic Ballet Club. Fergusson then spoke on the art side, saying we would arrange monthly exhibitions of members' work, and evenings of free discussion twice a week. Sir Patrick closed the evening on a note of optimism, welcoming me to Glasgow and wishing us all success in our endeavour to encourage culture in the city.

The results of that first meeting were encouraging, and we enrolled many members, enough to start the Celtic Ballet Club classes the following week. Among the first to join were Tom Macdonald, now well known as a painter and scenic designer, who lectures on art for *Adult Education*; and William Maclellan, the Glasgow publisher, who became a good friend and published Fergusson's book, *Modern Scottish Painting**. This book had been commissioned by Macmillan in London, but the war made the introduction of illustrated art books impossible. Maclellan, however, recognised its value as a contribution to Scottish art history, and had the courage to publish it without illustrations.

It was William Maclellan who took me to see the composer Erik Chisholm, who had been, and still is, sadly neglected in Scotland. He had composed several ballets on Scottish legends, and he played one of these to me, 'The Forsaken Mermaid'. I was enchanted by it, and saw that it was entirely suitable for presentation by my Celtic Ballet amateurs, most of the cast being fisher folk, so that the dances would have to be quite simple to be in character, and could thus be kept within the capacity of amateurs. The mermaids could be danced by my teachers and advanced students, and my choreography need not be too limited. Andrew Taylor-Elder agreed to design the costumes and scenery for this, our first production, which we planned for a year ahead.

Taylor-Elder was undoubtedly one of the most interesting artists of the period. He and Fergusson had met through the formation of the Ballet Club and had become great friends: but

---

* J. D. Fergusson, *Modern Scottish Painting* (William Maclellan, 1943)

they felt the Club was going to develop mainly on the theatre side, and that there should be a quite separate Art Club, and I agreed with them. Once again there was much discussion about a name. Finally it was decided that, as there was already an Art Club in Glasgow, always referred to by the young as the old Art Club, we would call ours the New Art Club: and at a meeting held at the Glasgow Art School in November 1940 this was agreed. We hired a large room over Jean's Tea Rooms in Sauchiehall Street, and held our first monthly exhibitions there. After a few months, however, we had to vacate these rooms, and, as we were by then unable to find anything central at a feasible rent, the exhibitions were held from then on at my school premises, rent free.

About this time I wrote to Sir John Stirling Maxwell, who had been one of our supporters since the spring of 1940, telling him of my hopes of creating a Scottish Ballet, and by return I received a cheque for £100 for expenses, though I had not asked him for a donation at all. I had, however, asked him if we could give a garden party that summer in the grounds of his beautiful property, Pollock House, with a performance in aid of the Celtic Ballet. He agreed at once, and asked me to visit him and view the gardens, which he put completely at our disposal for rehearsals and press photographs. We made good use of this, and I like to think we were able to make some return in the form of interest and gaiety for Sir John. Whenever we came to Pollock House he used to follow us around in his wheelchair, from which he watched everything we did with the keenest interest, providing us with soft drinks at frequent intervals, and begging us to come again.

When the day arrived it was one of typical Glasgow weather — just dull in the morning, turning to rain and then a steady down-pour in the afternoon. It really was heartbreaking; the grounds were so lovely, and our last rehearsal was given in full sunshine. Thanks to the excellent photographs taken by the press, the advance publicity had been good, and in spite of the wet weather about two hundred visitors did attend, including Sir Patrick Dolan, the Lord Provost: and all of them stood with umbrellas up to watch the performance, until the rain became a deluge and the dancers, with their costumes sticking to them and rain pouring off their head dresses, had to rush indoors for tea, followed by a stampede of dripping guests.

In December 1940 I took the Lyric Theatre in Glasgow, and put on 'The Forsaken Mermaid' in aid of the Glasgow Red Cross Hospital Supply Depot. Music and script, Erik Chisholm; costume design and décor, Andrew Taylor-Elder. It was the first big three-act ballet I had choreographed and produced myself, and there were many difficulties, dealing as I was mainly with amateurs; but I had Betty Simpson, who was wonderful as the Mermaid, and her fisherman lover Alan, Willison Taylor, though an amateur, was quick to learn, sensitive, and extremely good in the part. An orchestra in those early war days was out of the question, but we were lucky in that Erik Chisholm undertook to make a two-piano arrangement of his score, and Wight Henderson, the leading Glasgow pianist, agreed to play it with him. Obviously with trained dancers it could have been a great deal better: but, it was a really good show, and had a big success. We had several offers to stage it in other towns, but this was quite impossible with a largely amateur company over 60-strong, composed of doctors, lawyers, bank-clerks and so on, who could not leave their jobs even for a week. Nevertheless, in spite of all obstacles and drawbacks, I felt that my ambition of establishing a Ballet Company for Scotland might eventually be realised.

During the war years I put on three more important productions using amateurs in this way. These were:

1941: 'The Earth Shapers'. In aid of the Women's Voluntary Services. Music and script Erik Chisholm; costume design and décor, William Crosbie; choreography and production, Margaret Morris.

1942: 'The Ballet of the Palette'. In aid of Medical Supplies for Russia. Music, Stuart Findlay; conception, costume design and décor, Josef Herman; choreography, Betty Simpson.

1943: 'The Circus Family'. In aid of Glasgow Y.M.C.A. War Fund. Story and choreography, Margaret Morris; music, 'Sonata' by Eugene d'Albert; costume design and décor, Marie de Banzie.

For each of these productions, Isabel Jeayes came up from London specially to take charge of our publicity, and to supervise the making of hundreds of costumes, as usual on a purely voluntary basis.

In all of them, without drawing any invidious comparison, I was trying to follow what Diaghilev had undoubtedly been the first to do: to present ballets with first-class music, costume and décor, and choreography, and to weld all three artistic elements into a harmonious entity.

One of our most interesting productions was that of the fairy scenes from *A Midsummer Night's Dream*. Bottom was played by Stanley Baxter, now so well known on radio and television, who had started his training by attending classes at my school. He gave a remarkable performance. Oberon was Andrew Rolla, who after he left me was principal dancer in 'Brigadoon', and who is now directing the Movement classes at the Guildhall School of Dramatic Art. Odette Blum was Titania. The daughter of Hungarian refugees, she had been educated in Glasgow but was born in France, and though she could not speak a word of French she had to have a French passport when, later on, I took her on tour abroad. Puck was Thelma Bryant, a brilliant dancer, but I regret to say she eventually gave up dancing for the greater security of office work.

The décor was designed and painted by Donald Bain, a Glasgow painter, and was beautiful. I suggested large flowers to make the fairies look small. I designed the costumes and made them myself, with wonderful cooperation from my dancers. I cut up all my pre-war nightgowns and slips, which we dyed and edged with coloured tape to suggest the petals of flowers, and the effect was really very good.

Meanwhile, the students' training courses were going on as usual. The Western Infirmary were sending their physiotherapy students twice a week to our Maternity Diploma classes, and I was taking children's acting classes, as well as teaching dancing and painting throughout the school. We used to give end-of-term demonstrations at the Athenaeum Theatre, which is now part of the Glasgow College of Dramatic Art,

Dr Mavor, better known as the writer James Bridie, was a supporter of ours. He spoke at meetings and introduced several of our performances: but his interests were obviously on the literary and dramatic side, and I don't think art and dance meant much to him. During the performance of *A Midsummer Night's Dream*, when I was congratulating myself on the whole effect of lighting and décor, and the dancing of Oberon and Titania, I met James Bridie in the interval, and all he said was: 'I don't like your Glasgow children's accents!' I was terribly disappointed, because to me that was so unimportant. The children were training as dancers, and after all, was a Glasgow accent farther removed from the English of Shakespeare's day than that of an Oxford don or a BBC announcer?

I once produced a short play of Bridie's called *Saint Eloy and the Bear*. It is really a play within a full-length play, but we did it independently several times, for it was very successful. John Morton played Saint Eloy. He was one of the original Scottish National players, better known as Willie in the popular Scottish radio series 'The MacFlannels'.

James Bridie was a good friend to Fergusson, and was, I am sure, mainly instrumental in getting him elected as an Honorary Member of the old Glasgow Art Club. But Fergusson only went there once, and when someone asked Bridie why Fergusson never came to the Club he replied: 'Oh, don't you know? There are no women!' And that was quite true, for after the colour and variety of life of the Paris Cafés, filled with attractive, elegant women, Fergusson could not stand a room full of middle-aged men in dark suits.

Meantime I was trying to get the Scottish Education Authorities interested in my work. Dr Stewart Mackintosh, Director of Education, was always cooperative. He came to all our demonstrations, and seemed to appreciate what he saw. I remember once sitting next to him at a big display at the Kelvin Hall, in which many groups from colleges, keep-fit classes and so on were taking part. We had been allotted twenty minutes, and came on near the end. When our students ran on, and then did a few walking exercises, Dr Mackintosh turned to me and asked: 'How is it that your people run and walk with an easy grace that none of the others ever achieve?' To this I naturally replied: 'Because they are all trained on my method!' and then added: 'But they are in fact a very mixed group of various standards. I could make everyone run and walk and move generally with an easy grace and efficiency, though obviously some will move better than others.' He seemed impressed by this, and told me: 'I should like to get your method introduced into all our schools, but how? I cannot authorise new exercise classes without consulting the Department of Physical Education'.

As in London, I offered to provide teachers free for any controlled experiment in the schools, but, again as in London, this was refused. However, Dr Mackintosh was a man of great integrity and determination, and he asked me to come and see him and talk things over. When we met he told me the only schools over which he had a comparatively free hand were those for children with learning difficulties: and as I had already told him we had had some success with these, he asked me if I would like to try to interest the Heads of one or two of these schools. I agreed at once to see what I could do, and he gave me introductions then and there.

The Heads I met showed genuine interest, but as usual I had to offer to supply teachers free for a trial term, paying them myself. I did this at two schools, and the results were gratifying. Teachers of other subjects reported on the great improvement in coordination and also in concentration in the children who were learning my method. Many of those who had been unable to form letters were now beginning to do so. When the classes stopped the Heads were distressed, but I could not continue paying for the experiment indefinitely. I asked them to report on the success of the classes, and to ask for my health-play exercises to be included in the training of teachers for the learning disabled: but nothing ever came of it, and as this was only one of my many interests, I simply could not devote myself to the endless pushing and manoeuvring that seems to be essential for getting anything done on an official level in any new field.

All this time the New Art Club continued to thrive, and we had many interesting speakers at our discussions, including Dr T. J. Honeyman, who became Director of the Art Galleries and Museums of Glasgow, Dr Halliday, a leading psychologist, and Dr Friedlander, who became Director of Education in Israel after the war. But as always happens, some members grow dissatisfied, and resented the way the club was run and organised. One David Archer appeared. He had some money, and he offered to take premises in Scott Street, where a different kind of Club, to be known as The Centre, was presently formed. As I always believe in supporting any effort towards freedom in the Arts, I was one of the first to join and back this group: but I have found from years of experience that freedom in art can only be achieved through careful organisation of the practical details. When I asked Archer who was looking after the cleaning, tea-making, washing-up etc, he replied: 'Oh that will take care of itself. Anyone who happens to be around will do it!' My own experience is that no one happens to be around if any unpleasant job is to be done: and I was not proved wrong in this case.

The Centre got off to a great start. The lower room was decorated by Jankel Adler, the upper by Josef Herman, and an excellent exhibition of paintings was hung. David Archer provided a fascinating collection of art books, and we were all delighted about the venture. For the first few weeks enthusiasts gathered round, tidying up the place, making coffee and so on. But as all help was to be spontaneous, and as no one was to be responsible for seeing that anything was done, the first enthusiasm very soon wore off. No one made coffee or washed up any longer, the floors became filthy, crockery was broken or removed, and the art books simply disappeared, being borrowed without any record and never returned.

After about eighteen months of this, The Centre just faded out. This was tragic, because the premises and situation were perfect, and David Archer's ideas for the most part excellent: but my own conviction — that in order to have freedom in the arts you must organise the practical details of life — was borne out by the New Arts Club, which continued to flourish for twenty years. This was largely due to the fact that the practical side was dealt with by a small committee, who never interfered with the artists' freedom to paint and hang whatever they wished, or to express their opinions as frankly and loudly as they liked.

When the war ended we had a good number of M.M.M. students. Most of them were taking the educational and remedial training, but we had a few on the theatre side as well, including three young men, the most brilliant of these being Bruce McClure, who later became choreographer and producer for the Howard and Wyndhams 'Half-past-Eight' show in Edinburgh and Glasgow. As usual I was in search of professional outlets for this talented young group, and in the first few weeks of the post-war situation, a new project occurred to me. After the war certain towns in France had been 'adopted' by towns in Scotland. I had the idea of arranging a tour of these French towns, sending a small group of dancers with a piper and a Gaelic singer as well as the essential pianist. I discussed this with one of our New Art Club members, Captain George Girvan, a paratrooper and Resistance war hero, whose father was from Stirling, and mother from Abbeville. He was then teaching at Glasgow University; he arranged the whole tour, and accompanied the troupe as manager.

Betty Simpson was director and principal dancer. She did a movingly dramatic dance as Joan of Arc, to music by Bizet, which had a great success. As usual the audiences were tremendously appreciative, but the advance publicity had once again been inadequate, and I think it was at Orléans that the group arrived to find that neither posters nor newspaper advertisements had been displayed, so that scarcely a seat had been sold. I believe it was George Girvan's idea that our only hope was to parade through the town, the boys wearing kilts, the girls in the bright Highland costumes, the piper skirling away non-stop. This was done, and it succeeded in drawing a considerable and most enthusiastic audience. Many people came round afterwards, begging the troupe to return and declaring that they would pack the theatre; but sad to say, we have never yet been able to do so. Some day, perhaps?

The group returned to Scotland full of enthusiasm, for everywhere they went they had aroused great interest. In some places, members of the audience had waited to question them about Scottish customs and old legends, the origin of the kilt, and so on. The pipes of course, are closely related to the old Breton pipe, the *cornemuse*. The programme included two short ballets: 'The Hoodie Craw' for four dancers, by Erik Chisholm, and 'To Catch a Fish', for three dancers. The music for this had been specially written for me by Ian Whyte, then conductor of the BBC Orchestra in Glasgow. The script had been written by Winifred Bannister. This story was fresh and amusing, and was always a popular item. A boy is fishing happily, and when a girl tries to attract his attention he won't be distracted. He catches a fish, which he displays with pride. The girl snatches it from him. Now a gamekeeper enters and, seeing the girl with the fish, catches her up and walks off with her over his shoulder, leaving the boy in peace to go on fishing.

The Celtic Ballet Club continued to give monthly performances in Glasgow, not only of dances set to music, but also of abstract movements accompanied by poems. I presented several of Burn's poems in this way, largely in mime, but treated decoratively. It was about this time also that I expanded the dance to the music of the Skye Boat Song, which I had danced as a solo at the Celts and Scots Night, Queen's Hall, London, in 1939. This is a popular traditional song, not a great composition, but Bonnie Prince Charlie was a great rallying point in Scotland's fight for independence, and the song seems to me to symbolise the everlasting struggle, not only for political freedom, but for what is to me far more important, freedom of the spirit. I planned the dance for five women and four men. The men wore kilts and rough homespun shirts, the women long, simple, dark-coloured frocks, with large plaids in Highland tartans. These were used in different ways, spread out

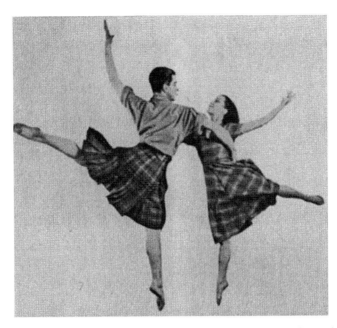

**The Celtic Ballet. 'Scottish Fantasia', 1954 (above);
and 'Skye Boat Song' (below).**

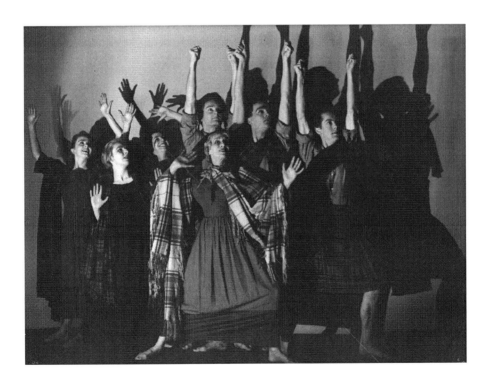

behind or wrapped closely round them, and finally waved triumphantly in the air. First presented at our Club productions, the Skye Boat Song was repeated at all our public performances afterwards, and it always brought the house down. I can claim it as my biggest choreographic success.

By this time our students were able to get grants for training with us, and we had a considerably number on the theatre side. During the Christmas holidays they easily got jobs dancing in the Howard and Wyndhams pantomimes. The producer, Freddie Carpenter, heard about my Skye Boat Song and asked me if I would like to include it in his *Goldilocks* pantomime, superintending its production myself. Kenneth MacKellar, now so well known as a singer of Scottish songs, was to be the soloist. I think this was his first appearance in a theatrical production. Freddie could not offer to pay me anything for the number, as his production budget was already complete; but Bruce McClure and the rest of my students who were in the show already knew the dance and were keen to do it: so I felt inclined to test it professionally in this way.

Actually I do not regret the time I spent rehearsing and attending dress rehearsals. Freddie Carpenter was a first-class producer, and his lighting effects were wonderful. He did not over-light as so many producers do now that almost unlimited light is at their command: and as he himself had been a professional dancer, he understood the lighting of movement, which is an art in itself.

I enjoyed having the entrée to any part of the theatre during the performance. I could go backstage and watch my number from the wings, or slip through the pass door to the front of the house, and see it with the audience from the back of the stalls: and if my dance was not up to standard, I would call a rehearsal. I could never get a seat, for the whole house was sold out for the season. One of the biggest thrills of my life was the reaction of the audience on the opening night of that pantomime, when that little dance of mine literally stopped the show. The audience clapped and stamped and shouted and would not stop! Of course it was a foolproof theme for a Scottish audience, but it proved to me that my dances could have a really strong popular appeal.

The success of this particular item was so obvious that it was repeated in the following year's pantomime. This again gave me the entrée to the theatre, and this time I put it to good use by making endless sketches backstage — some from the wings, some from the perches behind the spotlights, some from the flies. These, as at the Glasgow Alhambra, were still old-fashioned in those days, much of the scenery being hauled up on thick ropes by strong men. I made sketches of them too, which I sometimes gave them: and of course I drew from the front of the house as well. I painted several pictures from those sketches, in which the well-known Scottish actors Duncan Macrae, Harry Gordon and Jimmy Logan appear. I got to see the dance and ballet companies during the early Edinburgh Festivals by writing articles, with sketches, for the *Scottish Field*, which was great fun for me.

Suddenly I received a letter from Ted Shawn, asking me to come to his Summer School at Jacob's Pillow in the Berkshire Hills, USA, to dance and give classes in my method. In the thirty years that had passed since I first met him and Ruth St Denis in 1922, he had asked me more than once to come to America, but in the days when I had all my schools in Britain and France to see to, it was out of the question. Now that the war had cut down my activities drastically, it had become a possibility. It might even mean a start for a professional company. I wrote about it to Ted Shawn, suggesting that we bring a piper and a Gaelic singer, and show traditional Scottish dances as well as original ballets: and that Bruce McClure, besides dancing in these himself, could give classes in Scottish dance.

Ted was delighted with the idea, and at once made me a proposition. His school was called a University of the Dance, and students came from all parts to see, study and hear lectures on every type of dance, so he was able to bring us over on an educational basis. This meant we did not have to pay Equity-rate salaries, which are terribly high in the USA.

Ted Shawn guaranteed our expenses — travel, board and

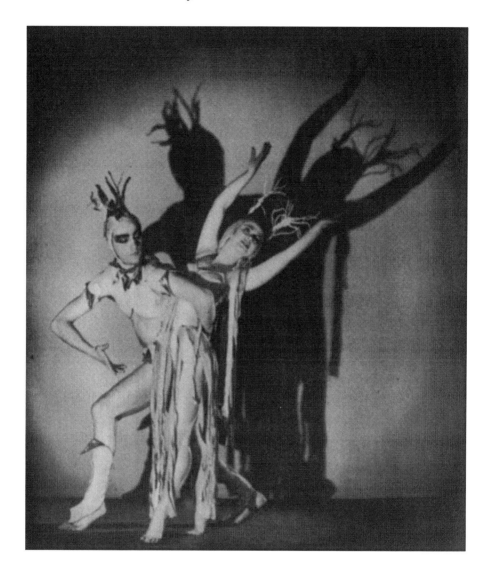

(Above) Bruce McClure ('Air') and Rena Steel ('Barley') in 'Barley Bree', 1954. Photograph: Scottish Studios.

(Opposite above) Jim Hastie (left) and Marie McGinn in 'Corn Riggs', 1961. Photograph: *Edinburgh Evening News*.

(Opposite below) 'The Deil's Awa', 1952. Photograph: Robert Anderson.

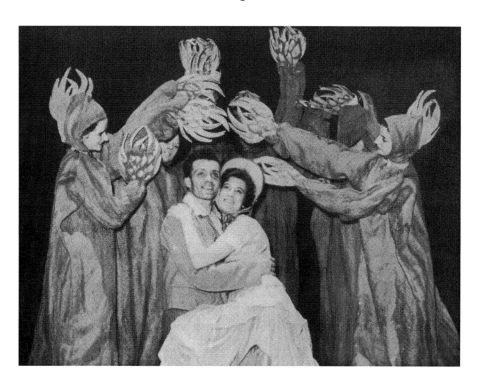

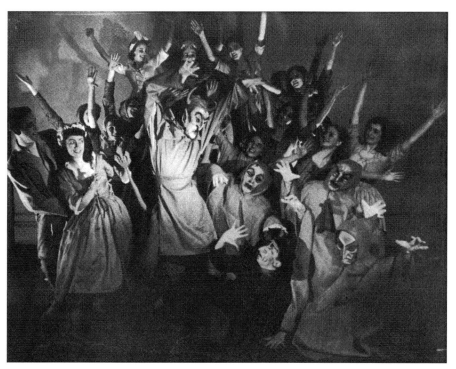

lodging — and provided pocket money for the whole company. Naturally, I had no difficulty in getting my pupils to agree to these conditions: they were delighted at the prospect of dancing in America. The Celtic Ballet was actually the first dance company to go to the USA from Scotland and this fact gained us a lot of publicity. I was very fortunate in being able to get Jack Skinner, my best male dancer, to come back to me for this engagement. He had been dancing for some time with the Ballet Jooss, but he now took charge of the company, and was wonderful at keeping them in order without being dislikeable. Sylvia MacBeth was principal dancer, as well as being in charge of wardrobe. This last was not an easy job, but she was a first-class organiser, and not even a shoe was lost throughout our visit.

The company was met at New York by a girls' pipe band, who came on board in the shortest of kilts, straight out of a musical show. Our piper was shocked, but the press were delighted, and took lots of photographs. It was my first taste of VIP treatment. The Americans certainly realise the importance of presenting their artists! Ted Shawn was a magnificent impresario. He arranged press and radio interviews, invited people to meet us, and gave parties after each opening night. We were there for three weeks, with three changes of programme, and were enthusiastically received. All our performances were sold out in advance, people crowded round us after each show, and the company had invitations to tea and cocktail parties almost every day. It was assumed that Scotch was our national beverage, so we were offered it at all times, wherever we went, to the delight of our piper and Gaelic singer, but not so much to mine, for their performances were not improved by too much American hospitality.

Ted Shawn insisted, quite rightly, that the boys of the company always wore kilts, as this made for good publicity when we went to any public place, where they were certain to be followed around and photographed. One of our boys was very shy and objected to this. Just before starting out for an important party given in our honour, he refused to put on his kilt. I was very worried until I suddenly had an idea. I sent for him and said: 'The

Americans admire the kilt, as you know, and they expect you to wear it as your national dress. Do you realise that if you are the only one in trousers, you will certainly be taken for the boys' dresser?' He put on his kilt without a word.

Besides being such a good impresario, Ted Shawn was also a charming and efficient host. Everything at Jacob's Pillow was well organised and well run, due also, of course, to the untiring efforts of his friend and co-director, John Christian, and to an excellent staff. We had a first-class pianist, Mary Campbell, who was wonderfully cooperative. The theatre itself is charming, and very well-equipped with lighting, drapes and everything else necessary. The entire back wall of the stage could be removed to show a natural background of hills, trees and sky, and sometimes the moon obliged as well. This made a wonderful setting for one of our ballets, 'The Road to the Isles'.

In spite of publicity and social engagements, we all worked very hard. We held classes every morning, fitted in rehearsals when we could, and gave performances every evening, except for the lighting rehearsal night, which I am glad to say Ted Shawn took very seriously and which he always attended in person. Following on our three weeks' engagement at Jacob's Pillow, he organised a short tour for us to summer theatres in New England, making all the arrangements himself. Accommodation was fixed for us everywhere, and we travelled in a huge bus, which took all our costumes and props. We were able to hang the frocks down the centre, so no ironing was needed on arrival. It was a wonderful experience to hear on reaching each new destination that the house was sold out in advance. Admittedly they were not very big theatres, but all were well equipped, and had efficient and cooperative back stage teams. I have never had so little trouble; all we had to do was perform. So often in my little Chelsea Theatre, I had to put up the scenery, fix the lighting, and even sweep the stage before the performance.

We shared the programme with the great exponent of Indian Dance, Ram Gopal; he demonstrated the language of the Indian Dance techniques, and did solo dances between our ballets. I thought it made for a programme of great variety. The traditional dances of India, the Highland and Scottish Country Dances, ballets on my free dance technique — all strikingly different, yet with much in common. Ram and I became friends; we used to watch all we could of each other's dances and we talked for hours comparing the different dance techniques.

The Indians, of course, use a lot of outward rotation and this has been likened to the ballet technique, but actually it is much nearer to mine, for the Indians start with the feet in the natural straight position for standing and walking, using the outward rotation of the hip joint when the knees are bent, or one knee raised to the side, or in stride position; exactly as I do, or rather I should say, as I do now, and as the Indians have done for thousands of years. Ram appreciated the similarities, and we thought how interesting it would be if we could dance together some day, to show how the two techniques could be blended.

I accordingly worked out the scenario for a ballet using my free dance technique but including the traditional dances of both India and Scotland, correctly performed. Ram was to dance the part of an Indian god. But our commitments have been such that Ram and I seldom meet, let alone have time to dance together. We are still friends, however, and perhaps some day our Indian-Scottish ballet may be realised.

I enjoyed every minute of that tour. I remember Maine, Kennybunk port and Vermont, where a charming hostess gave a party for us in her garden after the first show. The scenery was remarkably like that of Scotland, but everything seemed bigger and grander, with mountains, forests and waterfalls, even a full moon. It was an unforgettable experience: the warmth and spontaneity of American hospitality has to be experienced to be believed. Many charming women begged me to visit them for a week or two at their country homes; I could have spent months visiting, but I had to get back to Glasgow and my school.

The Glasgow press welcomed us back, and predicted a great future for the first Scottish ballet to invade America. But all that happened, as far as I was concerned, was that I lost my best dancers straight away and I could not blame them, for I had no immediate engagements to offer. Bruce McClure obtained a contract with Scottish television, and Andrew Rolla became principal dancer in 'Brigadoon'. Of course all small companies lose their best performers as soon as they are seen: but it was especially difficult for me, because I could not replace them from other schools, all my dancers being trained in my special technique, which took at least three years to perfect; and by this time the value of the American publicity had worn off.

I have kept contact, I am glad to say, with Ted Shawn. He and I were born in the same year, and we exchange annual photographs taken in bikini or trunks to show one another how young we are both keeping.

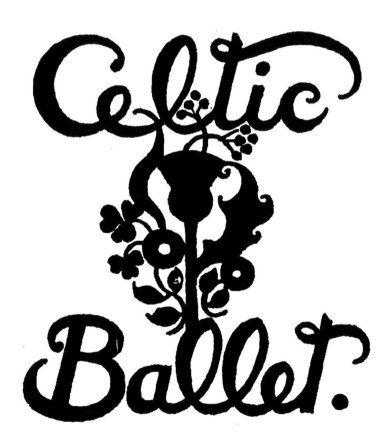

Celtic Ballet Design.

9

BY THE AUTUMN OF 1954 WE WERE ALL back again in Glasgow. The publicity from the American visit brought us more students on the theatre side, and Sylvia MacBeth was indefatigable in their training, for she shared my determination to establish a Scottish Ballet. Over the years I had had many interviews on this subject with Stuart Cruickshank, head of the Howard and Wyndhams Theatre Syndicate. He was always charming and cooperative up to a point, but he was afraid of launching my Celtic Ballet, believing that it might be regarded as too artistic or highbrow, and lacking in the necessary popular appeal. However, when we got the American engagement he was obviously impressed, and on my return I saw him again. He was still doubtful about our box-office value, and told me that in his opinion the name Celtic Ballet was not a good one. He suggested that I should change it to Scottish National Ballet, and this eventually is what we did, adding as a sub-title, A Folk Ballet — Traditional and Modern.

The change of name met with a good deal of opposition in certain quarters. In particular, the classical ballet schools were against it. They maintained that a national ballet must be based on classical ballet, but I did not myself see why the word ballet should be kept for one dance form only. The Ballet Jooss did no classical ballet, yet they had been touring under that name for many years without question. The actual word 'ballet' means 'a little dance', but it has come to have international standing in connection with a company of dancers, and I decided to use it for that reason.

The decision did not immediately produce an offer for a Howard and Wyndham tour: but in 1959 Kenneth Ireland,

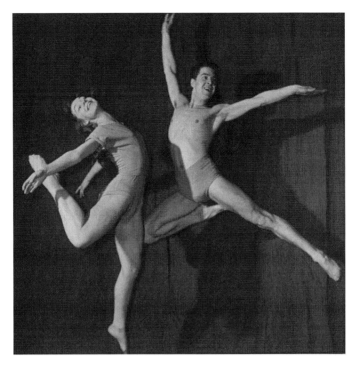

'Design and Action', performed for Scottish TV, 1959.

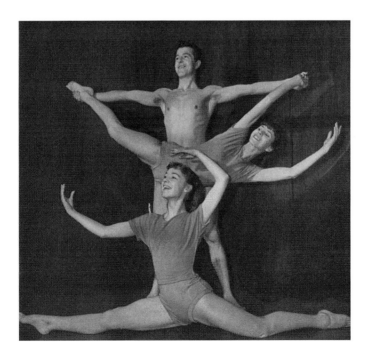

Director of the Pitlochry Festival Theatre, heard of my plan to launch a Scottish National Ballet, and offered us an engagement for one performance during the 1960 season. This was to be one of the matinées presented by dance groups, musical groups and soloists, which were, and still are, a feature of every season at Pitlochry: and I was delighted to accept.

We had a year in which to prepare our programme, and June 1960 saw our first performance under the name Scottish National Ballet. It was well attended, and the audience was enthusiastic, largely due to a wonderful backstage staff under the direction of Brian Shelton. It was a happy experience, and I felt it should be auspicious, for Pitlochry was the centre of the Highlands and the headquarters of the Perthshire Fergussons, my husband's clan, from which both his parents came.

After the show Kenneth Ireland presented me to Mrs Marjorie Fergusson of Baledmund, to her son, the Laird, Finlay Fergusson, and his wife Meg, all of whom have since become my friends. Marjorie Fergusson was delighted with our performance, and she talked to me about it with enthusiasm. She had been one of the most faithful supporters of the Pitlochry Theatre from its earliest beginnings in a tent, and she told me a great deal about those first days, when she used to lend furniture and put up various members of the company.

John Stewart, the founder, was an exceptional man, whole-heartedly devoted to the drama. To begin with he put all his money into running a tiny theatre in Glasgow, the Park Theatre. I gave two demonstrations there, but as the stage was only about ten feet across, what could be shown on it in the way of movement was very limited. Stewart then conceived the idea of founding a 'Theatre in the Hills', at Pitlochry. He had a house there, and he started the theatre in a tent, just like a circus, but it had a proscenium and lighting effects. Kenneth Ireland, who had worked with John Stewart at his theatre in Glasgow, went with him to Pitlochry: and when Stewart died in 1957, Kenneth carried on, and made a wonderful job of running and publicising the theatre seasons.

We left Pitlochry feeling encouraged, and I went to see Stuart

Cruickshank again, taking their programme with me. This time his attitude was far more encouraging. Evidently he now felt my ballet company really did exist at last! He looked up his book and said he could give us dates on quite good terms early in 1961, in Glasgow, Edinburgh and Aberdeen. I requested dates in England, at Newcastle, Liverpool and Manchester, where we had had such good audiences in the past. I pointed out that the pipes, the kilts, and the ballets based on Scottish stories would be a novelty in England; but I could not convince Mr Cruickshank, who seemed to think the financial risk would be greater over the border.

While all this was going on in Scotland, in London preparations had already begun for the Golden Jubilee of M.M.M. in 1960. The Directors had agreed in 1954 that a Jubilee Fund should be started, to raise money for a suitable celebration and a personal presentation to me. The trustees of this fund were Betty Simpson, Isabel Jeayes and Paul Beard. Isabel undertook the arduous work of organising, sending notices to students, past and present, teachers and friends. The response was most gratifying though mostly in small donations, and several teachers arranged dance shows and raffles to add to the fund.

In 1958 a Celebration Committee was formed with Lady Norton as President, and Angela Baddeley, Phyllis Calvert and Eleanor Elder as Vice-Presidents and Isabel as Organising Secretary. The Jubilee Week started on 17 October 1960, and the week's diary included an exhibition of photographs and drawings and paintings by pupils, press-cuttings books, and other items of interest from the files covering the first fifty years of the Movement. There was also an exhibition of painting by the M.M.M. Association Art Group of which J.D. Fergusson was the President and Nina Hosali the secretary. On Saturday 22 October, there was a demonstration of M.M.M. of all standards, and dances, at Cecil Sharp House, by pupils and students from all over the country; and in the evening a reception was held at 55 Park Lane.

Over a hundred and fifty gathered there from all parts, many from abroad. It was a wonderful party, with many joyful reunions. Some pupils had not met for thirty years or more. For me it was a most memorable evening; all around me people rose up out of the past to greet me, and some had come long distances; I felt surrounded by goodwill and love. I was especially pleased to see Philip Richardson, so long editor of the *Dancing Times*, for although he did not agree with my views on classical ballet, he was always fair, often giving us good notices and praising much of our work.

Phyllis Calvert made the presentation, and the way she spoke charmed everyone, she was so natural and spontaneous, recounting how she first came to my school, which I have told in a previous chapter, and paying a great tribute to my mother and myself for her training. The gifts I received left me speechless — unusual for me. Of course I was obliged to say a few words, but had to use all my willpower not to break down. Naturally, I had known about the fund, but the details of its progress had been kept from me, and knowing that not many of our pupils and friends were really well off, I only expected a token presentation. So when Phyllis handed me a cheque and share certificate amounting to over £500, I nearly passed out. There was also a beautiful little travelling clock in an emerald green case, a bound volume of our M.M.M. magazine, and last, but most certainly not least, a loose-leaf book of personal memories and messages, many with photographs from dozens of my teachers and pupils. This last was entirely Isabel's idea. She had invited contributions from every teacher and pupil she could find through old records. This book will always be one of my most treasured possessions.

But to get back to Scotland, I managed to fix a week at Carlisle for the Scottish National Ballet prior to our Glasgow booking. I knew we were sure of a good reception, because classes there were flourishing, and many enthusiastic supporters of my Movement lived in that town. Among these was Leila Shaw who had trained in my work in London and Glasgow. Her husband, Headmaster of Stanwix School, Carlisle, arranged for her to take classes in his school. She also won the support of the education authorities.

Meanwhile I had obtained, through an agent, a few more bookings in England to follow on after Aberdeen. I realised of course, that I should need some capital to launch this venture; but since it was obligatory to book a year ahead, I had to take the risk of accepting the Howard and Wyndhams bookings, and of signing their contract, before I knew where the money for the production was coming from. As soon as everything was definite, however, I issued an appeal for funds to found a Scottish National Ballet, and to finance the first tour.

Among those who helped most generously at various times were Sir Harold and Lady Yarrow, Lord and Lady Bilsland, Lady French, Lady Warren, Lord Inverclyde, Mrs Tombazis and Mrs Norman McCombe. Thanks to them, to many other generous contributors whose names I am sorry I cannot now remember, and to the hundreds of small donations from pupils and friends, we raised just on £2,000.

My theatre friends said I was quite mad to think that I could equip a ballet company and send it on tour on that amount. How right they were was proved by subsequent events: but of course I was relying on the fact that a good many of our ballets had already been produced, so that new décor and costumes did not have to be provided. I had reckoned, however, without Equity, the Actors' Union, a most necessary institution as I knew very well. As a child I had belonged to the Actors' Association, Equity's forerunner. But before that, performers had no protection whatever. A company could be stranded anywhere, and left to walk home, the management having closed down without warning. Nowadays that cannot happen, because every company must declare its salary list and lodge two weeks' salaries with Equity before a tour begins: and this sum is not returned to them until they put up two weeks' notice on the theatre notice-board, thus ensuring that all members will be paid. Since our weekly overheads, including salaries, fares, carriage of scenery etc, came to close on £500 — not much for a company of twenty-five, with a solo singer, piper and two pianists — there at once was our first £1,000 accounted for.

My next shock was to discover that the minimum rehearsal

salaries had been raised, just that year, from £4 to £9 weekly. For three weeks' rehearsal that took up another £600, leaving only £400 for additional costumes, and renewal of props and of scenery. Of course it is right that rehearsals should be paid for. Before the days of Equity a company might rehearse for three weeks without any payment, and the play might then be taken off at the end of the first week's run. But I do feel there might be some allowances made for small companies trying to do work of a cultural though uncommercial sort. Most of my dancers lived in Glasgow, and would have been willing to rehearse without salaries, but they were not allowed to do so. I was told that in America artists were not allowed to design scenery or costumes without payment. If that had been the rule here, my ballets would all have been done in the nude. I never paid anything to any of the artists who designed costumes and spent hours of their time making and painting scenery and props. Nor did they expect it. Although in my productions, the dancers were often not fully trained, so that the standard of performance fell far below the one I was aiming for, the décor and costumes were first-class and of great variety, because they were designed by real artists who watched rehearsals and cooperated in every way to create an aesthetic whole.

I was glad when Jack Skinner responded to my appeal to act as producer for the three weeks' rehearsal period, which he was able to fit in between his own engagements. He was indefatigable in his efforts, and succeeded in coordinating a very motley crowd. As a natural consequence of the American and Pitlochry engagements, several of my dancers, boys as well as girls, had recently been offered jobs in American musicals, TV and cabaret. For the first time, I had to advertise and hold auditions to recruit new dancers for the tour. The newcomers were trained in classical ballet and in nothing else, for at that time the American dance invasion was hardly under way, and the ballet schools all refused to allow their pupils to do 'modern American' while training, as it would spoil their style. Nowadays I doubt if there is any ballet school which does not include classes in modern American.

I eventually found four girls and two boys who seemed eager to join us, and to try to adapt themselves to my style of movement. They were all very cooperative, and in character numbers, or anything with sharp precise movement, they were quick to learn and did well: but they were incapable of achieving an easy flowing movement, or a simple, natural gesture. The harder they tried the worse they became; they simply could not help falling into the conventional ballet gestures and poses.

I was fortunate in finding an excellent Stage Director in a young chemist, Robin Anderson, who had come to me some years before in Glasgow. He told me then that he had been a Scottish champion skater, but that he had always wanted to dance, and was interested in what he had heard and read about my Celtic Ballet. He wanted to train, but as he had a full-time job he could only come to me over several years for private lessons. Nonetheless, he took part in many of our Celtic Ballet Club shows, and also proved himself exceptionally able at fixing and carrying out lighting effects. I learnt that he was intensely interested in the production side, and when I started the Scottish National Ballet, I engaged him as our Stage Director. He came with us to Pitlochry, and proved himself invaluable on our brief Howard and Wyndhams tour, taking part in some of the items, notably in the Skye Boat Song, in which I too danced. Robin Anderson was just behind me, and I enjoyed working with him; the fire and enthusiasm he generated was inspiring.

My principal male dancer was Jim Hastie, who had trained as a full-time student, and was an assiduous worker, always enthusiastic and cooperative, so that he made amazingly quick progress both in M.M.M. and in Highland dancing, which was now part of our curriculum. The principal female dancer was Sylvia MacBeth.

The programme consisted of the following ballets, together with traditional Scottish dances and songs with movement:

'The Harvesters : script, Marian McNeill; music, W.B. Moonie; choreography, Sylvia MacBeth; costumes and décor, Millie Frood.

'The Road to the Isles': script, Margaret Morris, music, traditional songs arranged by Kenneth Dawkins; choreography, Margaret Morris.

'To Catch a Fish: script, Winifred Bannister; music, Ian Whyte; choreography, Margaret Morris; costumes, Sheila Neill.

'The White Moth': old Scottish legend; music, Marie Dare; choreography, Veronica Bruce; costumes, Anne Young; décor, Donald Bain.

'Gods in the Gorbals': script, Margaret Morris; music, Kenneth Morrison; choreography, Margaret Morris and Bruce McClure; costumes, J. D. Fergusson and Margaret Morris.

The company was not big enough to present the larger ballets previously mentioned.

During the final rehearsals I had the devastating shock of the totally unexpected death of my husband, ending a forty-seven years' happy partnership.

And then, just before our tour opened, Howard and Wyndhams transferred our Glasgow booking from the King's Theatre to the Alhambra. This was a severe disappointment, for I knew we could have made a far more successful start at the King's, which is about half the size of the Alhambra. I had played at the King's many times, and looked forward to working there, for it is an intimate theatre, whereas the only good thing about our week at the Alhambra was the fact of my knowing the backstage staff through various pantomimes.

All the Alhambra staff were cooperative and friendly, and they did everything in their power to help us: but they could not help with the front of the house, and an audience that would have filled the King's Theatre gave us a depressing, half-empty house at the Alhambra. I dreaded the handing in of the receipt slips each night, for it soon became obvious that our sixty per cent would not give the £500 necessary to pay our salaries and other outgoings at the end of the week, and that I should have to overdraw to cover them.

During the second week in Edinburgh, business improved considerably, but we still did not take enough to cover expenses in full, and I had to overdraw again. This meant that I was faced with the horrifying problem of when to put up the fortnight's notice on the theatre notice-board. I had only signed Howard and Wyndham's contracts for the next two weeks in Scotland, but I had several subsequent weeks booked in England. All members of the company were on contract for the duration of the tour: but as soon as the fortnight's notice is put up, they are naturally at liberty to fix up whatever engagements they can secure. Should I risk the bank's allowing me a further overdraft to cover possible losses during our third week in Aberdeen? Or should I put up the notice at the opening of the week, to enable me to recover the £1,000 Equity deposit?

I wish now that I had risked it. The Aberdeen takings were better than Edinburgh's, and would have just covered our salaries: but the bank would not continue letting me overdraw without a guarantee. So I put up the fortnight's notice. My principal dancers at once booked up television shows, for which they were getting numerous offers as a result of the tour.

For our last date, in Sunderland, we had really good houses, as I had prophesied would happen in England. In Scotland, the highbrows thought a Scottish National Ballet sounded too popular, and the lowbrows wanted Scottish comedians, and thought we would be dull. Actually the lowbrows who did come were delighted, and I am convinced that, if we could have continued, we would have become successful.

This was proved by our reception in Sunderland, where we had full houses — even better, the box office told me, than Tommy Steele the week before! I expressed my surprise and was told: 'It's a novelty, you see. People ask if you have pipers, and wear the kilt, and they come out of curiosity.' What could I do, as my principal dancers were already booked for TV, but cancel the subsequent dates? I think the dancers were almost as sorry as I was.

10

THE TWENTY-ONE YEARS I SPENT living and working exclusively in Glasgow were the most exciting, the most satisfying, and yet the most frustrating of my whole life.

When, at the outbreak of war, six of my seven schools closed down, I found comfort in the thought that I was suddenly freed from the endless harassment of organisation and of examinations at all these schools, and I hoped that, with only the Glasgow school left, I might at last have time to create and produce new ballets, and perhaps even dance again myself in some of them: and to a great extent this hope was fulfiled. The Glasgow period was the most strictly creative I have ever known. During the war years I choreographed, for the first time in my life, really big ballets with forty to fifty performers. The frustration lay in the fact that these performers were nearly all amateurs, and that the ballets were only presented at single performances, which were given in aid of war charities.

Ever since the 'Celts and Scots Night' in 1938, at the old Queen's Hall in London, when Kitty MacLeod came from Scotland to sing in Gaelic, and I improvised dance interpretations to some of her songs, I had wished to prepare a programme showing the wealth of cultural material all over Scotland and the Isles: and at last I was able to do this in Glasgow.

The first thing I did was to arrange dances to the pipes for men and girls, the men in kilts with soft blue shirts, the girls in wide-skirted tartan frocks. (I never allowed the girls to wear the kilt as it is, and should remain, essentially a male garment.) The movements, though carefully thought out and designed, were

128

free and joyous, in contrast to the Highland and Scottish country dances, so controlled and restrained, as they have come down to us today. Attractive as they are, I have always felt that these dances in no way suggest the independence and freedom of spirit so characteristic of the Celts, which I have tried to convey.

Next I turned to songs of the Highlands and the Isles. I already knew 'The Songs of the Hebrides', Mrs Kennedy Fraser's inestimable contribution, and for the Lowlands I turned to the poems and songs of Robert Burns. This work was highly rewarding. I was already planning ballets for a company of fifteen to twenty, and dreaming of showing the culture of Scotland to the world. But here again creation led to frustration, for nearly thirty years later, apart from a fraction of Scotland and New England, USA, the world has not heard of us, and Scotland still means to most audiences only pipe bands, tartans and whisky.

After a year or two of working on these themes, I did the script, choreography and costume designs for a Burns ballet, which I called 'The De'ils Awa!' For this I arranged a sequence of songs and two poems, ending with the title song, which describes how 'the de'il cam fiddling through the town, and danced awa' wi' excise man!' The excise man was the official who confiscated illicit stills for making whisky, so it was a popular theme, with good comedy, and it was always applauded enthusiastically. The costumes belonged to the Burns period, making a change from the kilt and the tartan I was using so much.

I also evolved a ballet to a sequence of the wonderful Hebridean songs and tunes, of which there are so many, and I included a popular and beautiful song of Harry Lauder's, and named the ballet after it: 'The Road to the Isles'. The music was cleverly arranged by our conductor and chief pianist, Kenneth Dawkins, a great musician and a tireless worker. The ballet could be of any period, and I set it in the present day, with a party of young hikers singing round a camp fire and dancing to 'peut a beul' (mouth music). It was romantic, with a dream sequence and mist-maidens, but the music was haunting, and the whole ballet called for my naturalistic technique and continuity of movement. I have already told of the frustration I felt in this connection, when I had to use several dancers trained in classical ballet, who could not achieve a natural-looking movement.

Another satisfaction I had later on in Scotland was the creation of a really modern ballet, the idea for which came to me after seeing a ballet called 'The Gorbals Story', danced by the Sadler's Wells Ballet. It dealt with slum life in Glasgow, and it had a slightly sanctimonious strain I did not like: but it was dramatic and effective, and a forerunner of 'West Side Story'.

I wanted to do a ballet which suggested that the spirit of the Celts still exists, and comes through in the most unexpected places, so I chose the Gorbals — at that time still one of the toughest slum quarters in Glasgow — as my background, and called the ballet 'Gods in the Gorbals'. The entire area has now been almost completely transformed into up-to-date twenty storey blocks of flats, so that the title is already out-dated, and can have no meaning outside Glasgow. If the ballet is ever revived I shall re-name it 'Enter the Gods', or 'The Gods are Here!', the gods in question being of course the Celtic gods.

The scene is a typical backyard, with washing lines stretched right across the stage, with sheets, shirts and other laundry hanging on them. It is twilight, and a young girl is sitting on some steps leading to an open door, completely absorbed in a large book of Celtic legends. It is Hogmanay and her young man and a crowd of friends come rushing in with masks and lanterns, and try to draw her into their revelry: but she refuses and stays on alone, reading by the light from the door behind her. As the stage grows dark there appear on a large sheet, centre stage, the shadows of four figures, whose arm movements suggest Indian sculpture. The girl rushes forward and pulls down the sheet, revealing a glittering group — a god, a goddess, and two attendants. The girl is entranced: the Celtic gods exist — they are here! She calls her friends to come and see and they rush on from all sides with screams of delight, thinking the gods are just neighbours, dressed up for Hogmanay. They start dancing (jazz or jive) and eventually the gods are drawn in. The male god dances wildly with the girl, who is mesmerised, but when he sees the goddess enjoying herself with the girl's boyfriend, he becomes enraged, and puts a spell on all the mortals, so that they can only move to his command.

When the spell wears off the gods have vanished, and only the girl remembers them. Left alone with the boy, she will not look at him, but frantically pulls down all the sheets till the stage is empty. Then, sadly, she lets the boy lead her up the stage and through the door. The idea that I was trying to convey in this ballet is that the gods stand for the ideals and aspirations that are still with some of us, but that only a few people are aware of.

Nineteen sixty-one, with the totally unexpected death of my husband and the end of my ballet company just as it had achieved a box-office success, was the end of a chapter for me. I had to make a new start, alone. Although I was seventy, I had no intention of retiring, or of giving up striving for recognition of my claim that a complete method of training existed, other than the classical ballet, for forming creative dancers. I felt, however, that I must be free to travel as necessary, and because my training school inevitably tied me to Glasgow, I closed it. I have kept my flat up there, with many of my husband's pictures, and that is still my home, although I also share a London flat. In the summer I dive into the Mediterranean and lie in the sun, for I love France as much as I love Scotland.

London, when I first came back to it, did not seem to be encouraging as regards M.M.M. There were no headquarters and no training school. After the war Betty Simpson and Anne Cornock-Taylor, who had been working with me in Glasgow, had returned to London, where they took a large studio and ran a part-time training school and many outside classes. They also re-started the traditional M.M.M. Summer Schools: but this last centre of my training in London broke up after Betty's death in 1961. Meanwhile Isabel Jeayes, who had been my personal assistant for eight years before the war, had been storing and looking after the M.M.M. records ever since the outbreak of war had forced us to give up our lease of 31 Cromwell Road. (It was later destroyed by a bomb.) She had also stored certain costumes and properties, together with my personal files and effects. In this way it was Isabel personally who had become the essential support and centre of the M.M.M. organisation: and she was able to contact many of my ex-pupils and tell them that I should be spending half my time in London.

As time goes on I am amazed to find that my Movement, far from being dead, seems to be springing to life all around me. Many ex-pupils have been teaching classes and small groups in and around London, and several of my best teachers are running good connections in various parts of England, as well as abroad in France, Switzerland, America, South Africa, Canada and Trinidad. Acting in an honorary capacity as secretary and organiser, Isabel revived the M.M.M. Association. She was also responsible for re-starting the official Summer Schools at Taunton in 1963, Tiverton in 1964, Seaford in 1965, and at Bexhill in 1966. Monica Walter, one of our senior teachers who runs a successful connection in Sussex, helped with the organisation in 1967 and subsequently.

I am often asked why I don't start a Training College in London again, for we get many enquiries regarding full training, both from England and abroad. The answer is that I would do so provided someone else found suitable premises and took the full financial responsibility. I am ready to direct, teach and produce, for I am still young enough for anything I enjoy doing: but I am too old to risk having to worry about how to pay rent and salaries. I have done this for more than fifty years; from the age of twenty to well over seventy I have never been free of financial worries.

We are, however, still training teachers on an extended part-time basis. Authorised M.M.M. teachers prepare the students, and I then conduct intensive teacher-training courses at our Summer Schools and during the Christmas holidays in London. I have also conducted teaching courses in France, in the French language, for French and Swiss pupils who are now teaching M.M.M. in their own countries. The names of the exercises have been translated into French by Rita Prost, who was teaching for me in Paris before the war, and who, since her marriage to a

French judge, has been running M.M.M. classes and giving highly successful demonstrations wherever her husband has been stationed. I am hoping she will translate this book into French.

In 1968 the Central Council of Physical Recreation asked us to run a course in M.M.M. in April of that year, at their recreational centre near Torquay, and it was so well attended that we have been asked to repeat it. The CCPR — now a large and important body, with H.M. the Queen as Patron, and the Duke of Edinburgh as President — grew out of a small organisation called The National Council for Physical Education, which was formed in 1937. I was a member of its first committee, together with Prunella Stack, Lord Burleigh, Noel Baker, Mr S. Rous (now Sir Stanley Rous) and Mr A. H. Gem, the two last named being still on the Committee of the CCPR. The National Council started with the object of encouraging and providing facilities for recreational physical education and various forms of dancing: but with time its scope was widened, until it included every form of recreational physical activity — football, swimming, climbing etc. When eventually it became the CCPR, exercises and dancing occupied a very small corner of the organisational whole.

All my life I have acted on what I now realise was a misguided belief. This was that if I could actually show the results of my training method with children and adults of both sexes, as well as with people with learning difficulties and even the physically disabled, then the value of what I had to offer would become so obvious that the method would be officially recognised. But this never happened.

In March 1938 we took part in a demonstration at the Royal Albert Hall. This was a combined effort in which we joined with the English Folk Dance Society and the League of Health and Beauty. I cannot remember how it came about, but it was a very happy cooperation, and there were no serious disagreements. The three groups were so different in presentation that no invidious comparisons could be made. The Folk Dancers were already well known and accepted, and the black and white of the

Health and Beauty uniforms made a good contrast with M.M.M.'s blaze of colour. During the interval the three heads were presented to Her Majesty the Queen. I remember that some of my friends were shocked at my wearing the jade green coat I had worn for the demonstration and which was made of the cheapest cotton sateen! But Queen Elizabeth was charming and gracious, and I heard afterwards from Lady Buckmaster, who was Betty Simpson's sister, and who sat beside the Queen, that she had been delighted by our brilliant colours, and had also remarked on my 'beautiful speaking voice!' I had announced the exercises on a microphone, which was still something of an innovation, and I had been warned not to use my voice, which is actually loud and carrying, too powerfully, so I almost whispered into the mike, which seems to have achieved the right effect.

This was the first and biggest public demonstration in which we participated and we received a great ovation. I hoped some further cooperation with other groups might have been suggested, because I am a great believer in symbiosis, and am delighted when, if I have a success, others can share in it.

It seems to me that the dynamic people of the world, those who do things, or get things done, fall into two groups; first the creators and inventors, and second, the consolidators and the exploiters. I don't use the word exploiters in any derogatory sense, for both creators and consolidators are necessary if anything worthwhile is to reach a big public. Occasionally one individual may have both characteristics in his or her composition, and these lucky ones achieve success in their own lifetimes. But usually the creators, painters, poets and so on, are only fully appreciated after they are dead, and the real inventors earn little money while others, who are marketing the invention, earn much.

I belong definitely to the first group, but I have had to give the greater part of my energy to organising and dealing with financial problems, for which I know I am not in the least suited. The contribution that I have to make is the method which I have evolved, and which I believe to be the only one that really combines the aesthetic and remedial points of view. This is due to my having belonged to the art and theatre worlds before training as a physiotherapist. This has enabled me, over the years, to create a method of physical education, and a scheme of training, that produced teachers capable of passing on and making use of this duality, which is of outstanding value in dealing with both mentally and physically disabled people, as well as other children and adults.

Many of the things I fought for during fifty years are now accepted everywhere — bare legs, short, bright coloured tunics, and free expression in movement in all schools.

I am confident my work will be fully recognised and utilised once I am dead. I intend to go on working as long as I can for all I believe in, and I should like my epitaph to be the last lines of a bawdy song about a tart in the Klondyke:

But she died game boys,
Let me tell –
And had her boots on
When she fell –
So what the hell, boys –
What the hell!

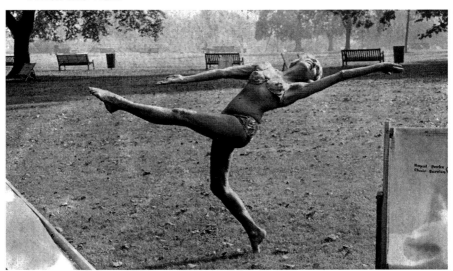

Margaret Morris practising in Regent's Park, 1965
Photograph: *The Evening Standard*.

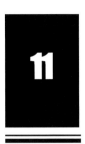

11

I WILL TRY TO GIVE AN OVERALL PICTURE of the M.M.M. technique, which I believe in its early stages provides a logical basis for all types of human movement, the reason being that we begin with absolute fundamentals — good breathing, posture, walking, running and exercises using natural movements. Only in its later stages is the technique developed and elaborated, or modified in various ways, to suit all types and ages.

Besides breathing and general exercises, limbering and stretching exercises are part of the daily practice. A supple body with full possibilities of the outward rotation of the hip joints is essential for stage dancing, and helpful for athletics and games; modified limbering is good for everybody, especially after middle age, because the tendons, particularly the flexor muscles, lose much of their elasticity and tend to contract and shorten.

We use no apparatus whatever; the ground or floor provides all the resistance necessary for stretching. For elderly and disabled people, who cannot easily sit or lie on the floor, limbering is done sitting on ordinary chairs, and for the severely disabled and the aged, there are special armchair exercises, which include very gentle limbering.

Throughout the technique from A to Z in every branch, the basic principle of combining medical and aesthetic values is integrated. Every exercise is a composition in form, a phrase of movement, done to music chosen to suggest the feeling of the exercise and how it should be done, whether strong, light, relaxed or whatever. But besides the aesthetic content, all the exercises have definite physiological aims and psychological values, making them at once beneficial and satisfying to do.

136

Pupils and patients never seem to grow bored; there is always the incentive to progress to a higher standard, the exercises being carefully graduated.

There are eleven standards of exercises, Basic, White, Yellow, Orange, Red, Light Pink, Dark Pink, Crimson, Mauve, Blue, Emerald Green. Students wear tunics of the colour of the exercises they are learning, so that in a big class or a demonstration, it is easy to see at a glance what standard any pupil has reached. Also the groups of different colours are very effective, especially when doing group improvisation. Colour cards are given out to those who reach the required amateur standard which means the exercises must have been thoroughly learnt and reasonably well performed, but imperfections due to age or any disability are allowed for. Professional students automatically move up to a higher class as they pass their colour tests — Professional Standard — and are expected to reach the highest colour, Green.

As I have already pointed out, the aesthetic side runs through the whole movement, but besides the design apparent in all the exercises in each class, some time should be given to free movement, improvisation and dance composition. Apart from the obvious value to professional dancers, it is now recognised that this is of great value to people of all ages in order to free the personality, get rid of inhibitions, and develop initiative.

Of course the approach has to be varied to suit or to humour different types and ages. Broadly speaking, children love improvising and composing dances; but some like to be picked as leaders, while others are shy and must be allowed to follow in a group until they have gained confidence. Adults are usually much more self conscious and sometimes opposed to any form of free expression. For these, a good way is to let the class do an exercise they know, and then tell them they can improvise a version of their own, with the same objective as the exercise, whether balance, stretching, relaxation etc. Those who are too diffident to try can continue to do the original exercise, and it will not be too noticeable.

Another easy start is what I call 'mirror following'. In this the teacher improvises, following the mood of the music, which should not be too fast, either suggesting slow relaxed movements, or strongly held positions. The teacher faces the class, and they all copy her as if looking at themselves in a mirror. The progression is to call on one of the pupils to lead; children love this, they stretch up their arms and the whole class stretches up their arms; they kneel, and the whole class kneels, copying and moving with them. We have a great many ways of doing group improvisation. I will describe a few later when I deal with basic choreography. I want now to enlarge a little on the technique for stage dancers and athletes, for the objectives in early training are very similar. If I live long enough I will deal with the other end of the scale and do a book on 'Movement and Art for the Physically or Mentally Disabled', indicating the main differences in approach and application, because we have had great success with both.

In dealing with any type of dancing, acrobatics, sports or games, where movement may at any moment be pushed to the limit, a knowledge of the anatomy and working of the main joints of the body and the muscles concerned in avoiding strains, is essential.

For those who don't know and others who knew but may have forgotten, the elbows and knees are hinge joints; the knee joint should always work in alignment with the ankle joint. The wrists and ankles are mainly hinge joints, though capable of a certain amount of lateral movement, but undue strain should not be put on them when out of alignment with the elbow or knee joints. Shoulders and hips are ball and socket joints and so capable of circular movements. High kicks to the side, and leg circling at hip level or higher, can only be done with a good outward rotation of the hip. The turned out position of the feet used throughout the classical ballet technique must come from an outward rotation at the hip joints. All good teachers of ballet emphasise this, explaining that unless the turn out of the feet comes from the hip joints, a great strain is put on the knees and ankles. This outward rotation of the hip joints is maintained throughout the ballet technique until it becomes habitual, so that even when a stride forward is taken, ballet dancers step forward with the hip outward rotated, so that the foot is at right angles to the direction of the stride, the knee also turning out as far as it can. This is an unnatural position, putting a strain on knee and ankle joints; and I think it looks ugly and distorted. On the other hand, in a lunging step to the side, the outward rotation of the hip allows the knee to bend over the foot in perfect alignment.

The point I want to make is that, in modern dance, athletics or games, though the limit of movement in all directions must be maintained, extreme positions should not become a habit, only being used with intention when needed. In my technique the outward rotation of the hips is used while limbering up, from the start of the training, but is not used in the Colour Standards until the exercises of normal movements are perfectly performed. In the higher standards, exercises emphasising the outward rotation are learned, and others using both the straight and the turned out position of the feet, to give practice in quick adjustment from one to the other.

Skating is a perfect example of the knee and ankle joints always working in alignment, because they can't do anything else. It is only possible to progress in the direction in which the skate is pointing; if you lunge forward with the foot turned out, you will inevitably shoot off to the side.

Footballers must be able to turn a foot out sometimes to stop a ball, but they must kick with a straight foot, and it should noted in relation to the value of the Greek position in football training, that any strong kick must be balanced by an opposition movement of arms and shoulders. I have dozens of photographs of eminent footballers in positions that occur exactly in M.M.M. exercises. Tight hamstrings severely limit the kick. When I was working at St Thomas's Hospital, footballers were often sent in to have their hamstrings stretched under anaesthetic, followed by exercises to keep them supple.

A supple spine is obviously of great importance in dancing. In athletics and games an acrobatic range of movement is not necessary, but it is of vital importance to maintain the tone of the intrinsic muscles, as these are the great safeguard against strains of the back in sudden movements.

In the second part of this book I explain the movements of the spine in detail, also the anatomy and mechanism of the Basic Breathing, and the first Greek position for opposition, because the understanding of these is of the utmost importance in relation to the daily health routines. But they are of supreme importance throughout the whole technique; indeed it is the emphasis on breathing, spinal mobility, and opposition movements, together with the creative side throughout, that are the outstanding features of M.M.M.

Obviously many objectives are common to all methods of training, such as agility, precision, good balance, and elevation, and of recent years the importance of relaxation has been appreciated. Indeed, sometimes free swinging movements seem to replace controlled movement and sustained effort, which are just as necessary if a training is to be well-balanced and complete.

I feel very strongly about what form the training in balance takes. Learning to balance on a beam high above the ground, except for professional gymnasts for displays, seems to be a waste of time, having little relation to activities that take place entirely on the ground. M.M.M. balance training starts with the babies playing at being storks, simply transferring the weight on to one leg, sliding the other foot up the leg to the knee, and down again — then trying to hold the balance position from two to four beats. This is also the beginning of the first Basic Balance with additions, a stretching forward at hip level and slow lowering of the leg, with appropriate arm movements, and synchronised breathing.

Each standard has progressively more difficult and complicated balances, eventually combining turns and jumps, landing and balancing on one foot, to develop the power of quick recovery after being thrown off balance through the unexpected hazards in games or boxing. Learning to fall without injury, when balance cannot be retained, is also taught, and is as useful on the stage as on the playing field.

The strikingly good elevation of our students has often been remarked on and much photographed, and this has been achieved by free standing, knee bending and springing exercises, without any ballet barre practice.

Continuity and flow of movement is just as important in athletics and games as in dancing. A few people seem to develop it naturally, even when it is not included in their training, as can be seen in the case of stars of football, cricket, tennis, skating and athletics, where the higher the standard of performance, the easier and more graceful it looks. My contention is, that with a training such as I have described, the majority could be brought up to a much higher standard than they reach at present, and the endurance of even our Olympic athletes could be greatly increased by systematic practice of full breathing, and breathing synchronised with a great variety of movements as in the advanced M.M.M. exercises.

Finally, some tough training is necessary for athletics and games, but skipping and running is overdone, being a constant repetition of the same muscular activity; obviously the runner must run, and the swimmer must swim, but all would benefit from general health and suppling exercises, and controlled breathing, before starting strenuous training.

I have said repeatedly that the aesthetic side is integrated throughout the technique, but I want to emphasise that besides the aesthetic composition of each exercise, free creative movement in one form or another is included in each class.

Choreography and dance improvisation are big subjects, and I believe that the study of both is necessary for the full development of either, though the approach to each is fundamentally different from the other.

Choreography covers the whole range of dance composition, solo or group, and ballets small or large: in every case the work, whatever it may be, is thought out, composed and rehearsed, and should be consistent at each performance.

Dance improvisation on the other hand, as the name suggests, must always be completely spontaneous and unrehearsed; it should be the uninhibited response to music, drum beats, or words. I am not going deeply into the matter here, as the later stages only concern professional dancers, and would-be choreographers. But I will indicate how M.M.M. introduces pupils to these two fascinating subjects.

In approaching creative work in any type of dancing, a certain knowledge of the fundamentals of design are most helpful, and ground plans, grouping colour effects and costumes can all be worked out on paper. Certain facts are inescapable:

1. Every composition, however, free, is inevitably limited by a certain space; in painting, the sheet of paper, the canvas or a wall; in theatre, the stage, or floor space if in the round. Even a pageant field must end somewhere.

2. All compositions in painting or movement are either *(a)* symmetric, *(b)* asymmetric, or *(c)* a mixture of both.

3. All effects are arrived at through *(a)* similarity of movements, designs, colours etc, *(b)* contrasts of movements, designs, colours etc, or *(c)* a mixture of both.

The degrees of each and the variety of treatment are infinite. I have indicated as it were the skeleton on which a composition can be built. No formula can create a work of art, but from the study and appreciation of basic principles, sometimes a real work of art may emerge.

Dance Composition

We begin with 'group building', using from four to eight in a group. This is done in two ways: *cooperative* — each person taking a position they think will add to the composition as a whole; or *individual* — one person arranging the whole group. The teacher dictates whether the group is to be symmetric or asymmetric and may suggest a subject such as fear or joy. When dealing with beginners it is easier to start by limiting the groups to simple lines, whether straight or curved. To practice 'similarity' and 'contrasts', we divide the class into pairs, one pupil immediately behind the other. The one behind either copies and moves with the one in front, or moves in contrast. Ground plans are explained and worked out with the class.

Eventually, a class dance is arranged cooperatively. For individual composition it is best to begin with a duet or a trio, solos can be composed for practice but are seldom good enough to be put into demonstrations; duets and trios can always be made interesting even with indifferent performers, if the movements and groups are well designed.

Dance Improvisation

Free movement and improvisation to music are now generally accepted in education, but their interest as an artistic spectacle has yet to be demonstrated. Musically, dance improvisation falls into two sections:

1. The dancers endeavour to interpret the music played (which may be composed pieces or improvised playing).

2. The dancers having been given a subject, idea or situation, convey it in their own way; the music, which in this case must be improvised, follows the mood of the dancers. This calls for good dancers with imagination as well as technique, but is of less interest musically.

Years ago I evolved a partially organised way of improvisation. This sounds contradictory, but it in no way interferes with the freedom of the dancers. We call it group improvisation. There are literally dozens of ways of doing it, to which several of my teachers have made valuable contributions. I have already mentioned 'mirror following'. We also have 'simultaneous following' and 'delayed following'. In each case, it is only the leader who improvises, the rest following. This is useful in getting diffident people started, since they merely have to copy the leader.

There are many other ways of doing free movement, but with an organised ground plan, or organised starting positions. The second stage of group improvisation is entirely free, though this calls for well-trained musical dancers used to working together. Much of this only concerns dancers, and the whole subject may not seem to have any great relation to athletics and games. But actually I am convinced that the study of cooperative group building, ground plans, and an appreciation of design in the placing of individuals and groups, develops qualities decidedly useful on the playing fields.

I have been re-reading what I wrote over fifty years ago, published in my book *Margaret Morris Dancing*[6] illustrated with Fred Daniel's photographs. I think it is entirely relevant to the present day, though I appear to have been a terribly earnest and serious young woman! With all my other activities, it took me years to write that book, and I seem to write more light-heartedly at seventy-seven than at twenty-seven. I am glad to find however, that I agree with everything I said in this early book: and I feel I must quote here the chapter dealing with my ideas on the training of creative dancers, urging the study of form, line and colour, all theatre production, especially ballets and dances, being mainly a visual art.

'I will first take the stage point of view, because it is the most obvious. Anything presented on the stage is a picture, a picture in a very definite frame. As you have no other sense with which to be aware of, or register impressions of movement, except sight, it is obviously a visual art, and, as a visual art, it cannot help being a combination of some kind of form, line and colour.

But whereas the painter is always trying to suggest movement and light, on the stage there actually are people to move, and light that can be changed many times in one picture or setting.

When one considers how far behind, artistically, any stage work is to any first-class painting, it makes one realise how little the possibilities of this wonderful medium have been explored. I am concerned in this chapter with the importance of the study of form and colour to the dancer and composer of compositions in movement — whether for the stage, for educational purposes, or for amusement.

If we admit that stage productions may be considered as pictures, then the dancers are part of those pictures, and the direction and shape of their movements of the utmost importance to the composition as a whole. The analogy between pictures and dances presented on a stage is fairly obvious, but it is also true of any composition of movements, wherever performed — a room or garden; for there must always be a limit to the size of the composition, and that limitation of space is to the dancer as the canvas to the painter. A dance performed in an open space is as a picture without a frame. The dance should be composed always in relation to this space limit, as a picture should be painted in relation to the size and proportion of the canvas, and designed accordingly.

It seems to me obvious that no interesting composition, satisfying to the eye, can be arrived at by stringing together set steps which serve only to show off the agility of the dancers, and have no relation to the picture as a whole. Many have realised that this is an absurdity, and that no dance composed in that way could possibly deserve any serious consideration as a work of art. But they have always turned to the interpretation of the music as a solution.

Certainly it is a very important point, but it is not the key to the understanding of composition in movement: because as I have said above, it is a visual art, and therefore must be studied primarily through the sight. Those who believe music and the understanding of it to be the true basis of 'the dance', think that by following the phrasing, and interpreting the music with movements that they feel to express it, they are creating a work of art: whereas though they may be feeling it intensely, if they have no knowledge of composition in form and colour, they cannot possibly know if the shapes and series of movements they are making are conveying to the spectators in the very least the emotion that they themselves are feeling.

A dancer who had very little technique as regards bodily agility, with an understanding of form and colour, could compose, and even perform, dances much more interesting to look at, as regards composition and interpretation of the music, than a dancer with brilliant technique but no understanding of form and colour.

Movement is the most primitive of the arts, and the most closely allied to our daily lives: therefore the understanding of it, not only through physical exercises, but through the study of the shapes and lines made in dancing, must be of great value. In our daily lives we cannot help moving in relation to our surroundings, to some objects or persons; and to a great extent, according to the harmony or disharmony of these relations, our lives become harmonised or disharmonised. The study of movement visually links up the physical and mental control of muscle and brain. Most people have never learnt to use their eyes, and a more general study of seeing and moving would lead to a far greater tranquillity and harmony of rhythm than we see around us at present.'

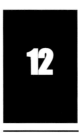

In 1910 JOHN AND ADA GALSWORTHY had insisted I must start a school and helped me to do so. They agreed that it was most important that I should try to evolve a notation of movement. Raymond Duncan had noted the arms of the Greek position, which was easy, as they were always done in profile: so to the arms I added signs for legs and feet, and started teaching this simple notation to my pupils. In 1913 this attracted some attention in the press. But I soon realised that to be capable of recording every kind of human movement, notation could not be pictorially representative, and I endeavoured to devise symbols that would be as abstract as possible. At that time I had not heard of the early methods, nor even of Nijinsky's: it is interesting to note that Laban, whose method of notation is the best known and most widely established today, was working out his method in another part of the world at the same time that I was working out mine in London.

Until 1920 my entire interest was in the dance and the theatre, so naturally I turned to the notation of music in evolving my notation of dance. It seemed obvious that, when working with music, it would be desirable to write the movements from left to right, with divisions into bars and time signatures. I drew a 'stave' with three lines for arms and hands and three lines for legs and feet, and a space in the middle for the body.

As all movements of arms or legs are either right or left, I thought it would be a great saving of time if no signs were needed for this: I decided to write all positions of the right arm or leg *across a line*, and all positions of the left, *under a line*. The lines and spaces are also used to indicate the *level* at which a movement takes place.

My next idea was that as arms and legs are attached to the trunk, they can only move in a circumference round the trunk, so if there are signs for *all directions*, to be written *at all levels*, it should be possible to record any movements. This works admirably for simple positions, but when rotations of the shoulders and hips are added, or that awkward articulation of the forearm, the radio-ulnar joint, then the troubles of the notator begin. But the foundation must be laid by taking the simple things first.

In choosing signs of direction, the first question I put to myself was: 'Which direction will be used most often?' Obviously progression is mostly forward — walking, running and hopping — and many arm movements are also in the forward direction. I decided that a forward movement should be represented by a single sloping line, the quickest and easiest to write. A backward movement could have been sloping the opposite way, but I considered in quick writing this might become confusing, so I substituted a straight line.

It then seemed to follow logically that movements sideways could be made up of the two. The diagram on page 147 makes this clear. For feet under you, or arms straight down or straight up from the shoulder, a perpendicular line seemed obvious.

In 1928 Kegan Paul published my book, *The Notation of Movement*, in their 'Miniature Psyche' series, but I have made several alterations and additions since. I have reduced the stave to four instead of six lines, using a dot when necessary to replace a line: and the way the levels are indicated is also different, and far more accurate. I began by taking the leg and foot levels in relation to the ground, as at least one foot is mostly on the ground, but I found this became confusing when lying down or doing a handstand. It was obvious that the only constant relationship for the arms or legs was to the trunk, and to each other. Therefore, leg levels are taken by the knee, as arm levels are taken by the elbow.

The position of hands or feet are determined by the degree of flexion in elbow and knee joints. In the case of the arms this

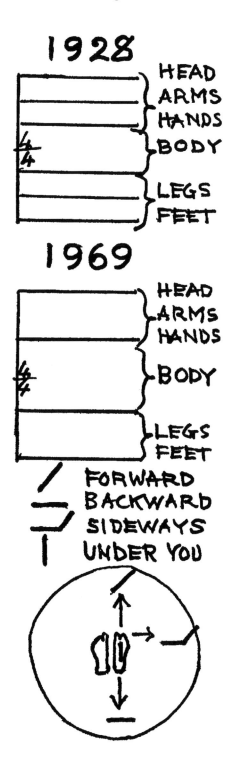

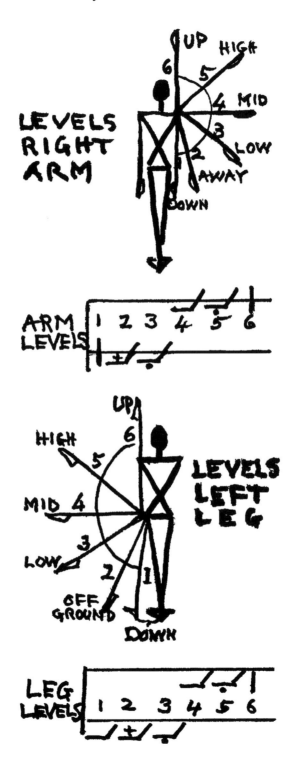

is complicated, as I have mentioned, by rotation of the shoulders and the radio-ulnar joints, and in the case of the legs by the hip-rotations. Flexions are written across the signs of direction. I have not space here to go into how the various degrees of flexions combine with shoulder rotations, nor the movements of ankle and wrist joints, which are all provided for. I am trying to give an overall picture.

The movements of the trunk and of the head are easier to describe because they are much more limited. I show this on the previous page.

Since 1928 I have altered my method of notating turns. In my book I use a small square, of which one side represented a quarter-turn, two sides a half-turn and so on. But though quite clear, I felt it was aesthetically wrong, as there are no sharp angles — nothing square in fact — about a turn. I will give the signs that I use now. Written under the stave the turns apply to the whole body, but they can also be used for circling of hands, feet, etc. (see previous page).

Lastly, transition and expression signs are of the utmost importance. It seems to me obvious that any notation of movement can in reality only notate *positions* and indicate *transitions*. A film is the only way of recording transitions perfectly, but a film, when stopped, is seen to be only a series of positions recorded at high speed.

It is obviously impossible for any human being to record movement at the speed of a film camera: therefore all one can do is to notate the main positions held or passed through, and indicate the way the transitions are to be done. These transition signs are tremendously important, so I give my main transition or expression signs overleaf. Of course the first binding sign is taken directly from the music.

Here I must mention Robin Anderson again, because he helped me considerably in the final adjustment of levels, flexions and rotations, and also prepared the material for transparencies sent to the Bureau of Dance Notation in New York, by whom we were invited, through Ann Hutchinson, to contribute material to be used in their lectures. She started a similar bureau in London,

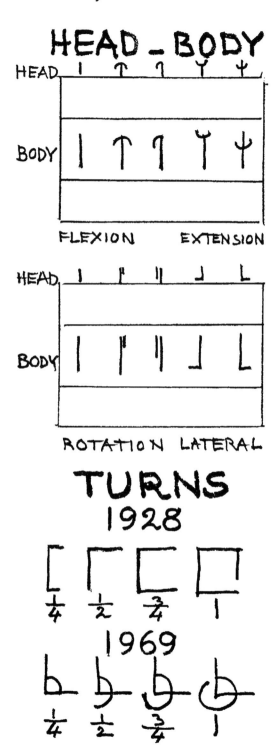

on which I was represented by Isabel Jeayes: but it seems it was not possible to continue it.

There has recently been a series of articles in the *Dancing Times* which has done a great service to the dance, and indeed to all forms of movement, by bringing this subject to the fore. A. V. Coton began it in the February 1968 issue when he discussed the three methods available today, Laban, Benesh, and my own. Ann Hutchinson followed up with three interesting and well-informed articles dealing with Labanotation and the Benesh Notation, and replies on the Benesh Method followed.

Obviously it is not for the creator of one method to evaluate the others: and I still hope that eventually some unbiased experts may be found to investigate and compare the available methods, including my own. Clearly only one method should in time be adopted as in music.

Before writing this chapter, I attempted to investigate — though only superficially — the Laban and Benesh methods. I borrowed a copy of *Labanotation*[7] by Ann Hutchinson, which is now out of print. It is masterly. I also studied an introductory book on the Benesh method, and after comparing the three ways of writing the same movements, I came to the conclusion that mine compared favourably with the other two. My signs are undoubtedly simpler and quicker to write than the Laban. The Benesh, on the other hand, are simpler and quicker to write than mine, but so small that I think they become confusing. Shorthand notes are adequate for recording long-established techniques such as classical ballets, Spanish or Indian dances, where the sequence and manner of performance are well known: but for recording creative dances and ballets, with really original and free movements, and also for medical work, a detailed notation is essential. It seems to me that the Laban method can record all details accurately. But I do not consider that the upright stave, writing from below upwards instead of from left to right, though satisfactory for the Chinese, can be the easiest for the large majority who write from left to right and who would use the notation in conjunction with a musical score.

The Benesh method, while it started out only to record ballet, now claims to have enlarged its scope to include athletics and all remedial exercises.

In her second article in the *Dancing Times*, Ann Hutchinson lists the ways in which the various systems should be examined, and concludes: 'Such study and research would require a grant to cover at least five years, probably more.' Is it is too much to hope that a start might be made in finding retired specialists in different fields, who would be willing to give their time to study the material supplied by the notation methods to be investigated, and to give their opinions on their respective values? Eventually a grant would be necessary if experts were required, and practical experiments carried out on the methods found worth of consideration. But need this take so long?

I would like the 'retired investigators' (if any can be found) to include: (1) a mathematician or scientist, with an understanding of symbols and signs; (2) a doctor, with experience of bodily movement; (3) a physiotherapist, to evaluate correct recording of remedial work: (4) an expert on physical education and athletics; (5) a musician, to evaluate the relationship to music; (6) a choreographer of both classical ballet and modern dance; (7) a producer, to evaluate suitability for recording for television and films.

Although I should like my system to be properly tested, I am objective about it, and am genuinely ready to discard it in favour of any other method that can be proved to be more efficient and practical than mine. This is because I am convinced that there should be only ONE METHOD OF NOTATION, capable of recording any human movement, and of being understood by any nationality. Any method of notation that exists today deserves serious investigation, for this is a subject that has been far too long neglected. In the recent Laban-Benesh discussions in the *Dancing Times* a good deal was written about the number of people now using or studying the various methods, and also the quantity of books and pamphlets available about each. It is the methods that should be evaluated, their capabilities of recording human movement, the ease with which they can be read, and the speed at which they can be written.

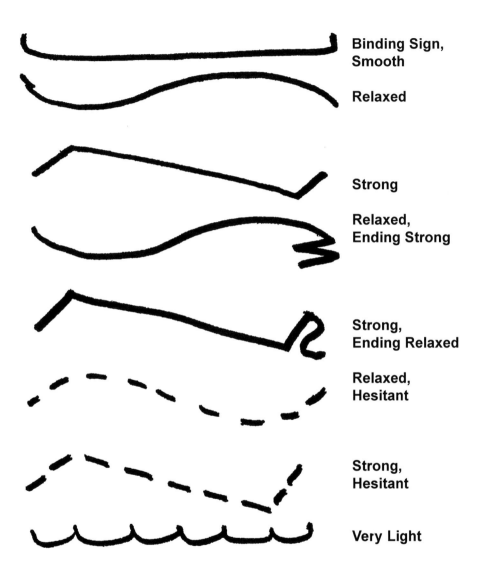

Binding Sign,
Smooth

Relaxed

Strong

Relaxed,
Ending Strong

Strong,
Ending Relaxed

Relaxed,
Hesitant

Strong,
Hesitant

Very Light

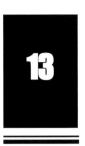

13

HAVING DESCRIBED MY MOVEMENT from birth to maturity, covering close on sixty years, I now want to say something about other styles of dance, and possible developments. It may appear from the previous chapters that I am interested only in what I am doing myself. Some of my friends reproach me with this, and I admit that to some extent it is true. I should never have created my technique of movement, or my notation of movement, if I had been too concerned with what others were doing. I am delighted to find a lot of experimental work in dance and lighting going on today. But don't they all seem to be working along almost identical lines? I have seen nothing as striking as Gordon Craig's designs, using blocks or drapes, with shadow-masses, and light.

The masters of the past should on no account be copied, but their work should be a stepping-stone to further creation. James Pride, to whom Craig owed a lot, was a real innovator, but Craig carried his work much farther, and it is Craig in particular who should be studied. His work has never been fully appreciated in his own country, and it could open up a new path of experiment. It looks modern even now. What originality and courage it must have taken to present his work, after the productions of Irving and Beerbohm Tree!

Sixty, or even fifty years ago, very little was being done here to further the art of dancing. No English ballet existed, and I don't think there were any schools of free work except mine. America was far ahead of us in the modern dance movement, mainly due to the Denishawn School, the first to make their pupils study various types of dance, and to present original dance works with their company which toured the USA.

It is not possible to be equally concerned with creation and research at the same time. Now that I am not so busy, I am most anxious to know what others have been, and are, doing. First I want to state emphatically that I am in no way opposed to the classical ballet as a specialised art form. I admire and enjoy it tremendously when it is perfectly done, and when the subjects are suitable for interpretation through the stylised technique and accepted conventions of the ballet. But I do object to the claim put forward that the ballet technique is the only possible foundation for every type of modern and experimental dance, and even for athletics, and I am ready to debate this with experts in all fields. Yet if I were asked to name the most perfect artistic stage achievement I have ever seen, I would cite Diaghilev's Russian ballet. My admiration was, and is, unbounded, and I am glad that I am old enough to have seen them when they first came to the Drury Lane Theatre. Karsavina and Nijinsky stand out in my mind above all, and of course the choreography of Fokine.

Karsavina is the greatest dancer I have ever seen, for besides having a technique brought to such perfection that one did not notice it, she was a superb actress. She seemed to live each part, endowing them with subtle differences, but always conveying a richness and depth of feeling.

Pavlova I also saw, and loved. Her lightness and ease of movement and personal charm were irresistible, but in my opinion she never reached the heights of Karsavina. I never saw Pavlova really well presented; she had a most inadequate company, and ordinary scenery and costumes, not helped by the complete lack of artistry in lighting. It must be remembered that it was Diaghilev's genius for picking the right artists, composers and choreographers, inducing them to work together and unifying the whole production with wonderful lighting, that presented the dancers as never before, so that Karsavina shone like a beautiful jewel in a perfect setting.

Nijinsky was exceptional as a dancer. He literally had legs like a grasshopper — the muscular development of his thighs being quite abnormal — and he was also a great actor. I can never forget the uncanny allure of the 'Faune', the frenzied passion of his slave in 'Scheherezade', and greatest of all, his puppet in 'Petrouchka'. His performance in this was simple, restrained, yet so sad that it seemed to typify the tragedy of life. I have not been moved in the same way since. But Nijinsky was not only a spectacular dancer: what to me was more important, he was a great choreographer, and he had the urge to break away from the conventional technique in which he excelled, and create new dance idioms, and he never mixed the styles. 'L'Après-midi d'un Faune' was pure archaic Greek postures, and 'Le Sacre du Printemps' was even more extreme, the toes being turned in instead of out, and throughout both ballets there was not a single ballet position.

In recent years I have often been distressed at the way ballet and naturalistic dance and mime are mixed, for no apparent reason. I admit styles can be mixed with great effect, as was done by Massine in his Scottish ballet, which I shall describe later. I am thinking particularly of some modern ballets, and abstract interpretations of music, which for the most part are simple free movements with interesting grouping or naturalistic mime in soft draperies, or leotards, and then suddenly, for no apparent reason, the principal dancers go through the most conventional ballet routines. One ballet that charmed me was a story of simple country people; the girls wore plain frocks to the ankles in soft dark materials; the choreography was first-class and entirely suitable to the theme, until suddenly, in the supremely tragic moment, the principal dancer did a solo on her points. I suppose to the balletomane the points express the height of emotion, but to the human being with more ordinary reactions, it just looks like exhibitionism, with no relation to the dramatic content of the story. All this saddened me, but the fault lies with the choreographers and the way they use the ballet conventions.

The achievements of pioneers in any field — those who have managed through hard work and persistence to break through — have always aroused my admiration, so I want to pay tribute to the two early pioneers of the English ballet, Ninette de Valois and Marie Rambert. It was in the 'twenties that Ninette de Valois started her school, later working in collaboration with Lilian Baylis. From this partnership there emerged the Sadler's Wells Ballet, which is now known as the Royal Ballet. Marie Rambert had also started a school and formed the Ballet Club, later to be known as the Ballet Rambert, which gave performances in the now famous Mercury Theatre. This became a forcing ground for modern choreographers, and her company produced many outstandingly original ballets. Undoubtedly these two schools were the foundation of British ballet as we know it today.

But what of those who broke away from the ballet conventions to create freer forms of dance? I think the revolution started with Isadora Duncan, was carried on by Ruth St Denis, and then spread to Germany where Mary Wigman (a pupil of Laban's) and Kurt Jooss evolved individual styles. As I have said America was far ahead of England in creative dance, partly because of the great mixture of races, and through them the many ethnic dance influences that are present in the USA.

The Denishawn School was certainly the first to recognise and make use of these influences. Martha Graham and many other creative dancers had their early training there.

Of the early revolutionaries in the 'twenties, I think Mary Wigman was the greatest influence. I never saw her, but one of my best pupils, Leslie Burrowes, left me to work with her in Germany. I was very sad about this, because Leslie was a lovely dancer, very supple, and with good elevation, and I hoped she would develop a dance style of her own. I always wanted my pupils to build on what I had given them, and carry it further. But Leslie went to Germany and came back with the Wigman technique of clinging to the ground. Gone were all her lovely leaps and free and joyous movements; it was all down to earth and stamping with flat feet. I admit Leslie had gained in depth of dramatic expression, but it was all so tortured and tragic and possessed no variety at all. I had hoped she would have assimilated the best from both methods. Soon after her return she married Leon Goossens, whom she had met some years previously at my Little Theatre and they now have two daughters, and Leslie no longer dances.

Kurt Jooss was one of the first to tour with his own company, presenting original ballets. His 'Green Table' is deservedly world famous, for it really is a masterpiece, and his 'Big City' was extremely good, and a forerunner to the type of choreography seen in 'West Side Story'.

A company I enjoyed tremendously when they came to Glasgow was Katherine Dunham's Group: they were all from diverse ethnic minorities. She herself had been a university student and had done research into ethnic dance, and most of the ballets depicted customs and tribal ceremonies, but some were quite modern, and there was much variety. Katherine Dunham had a charming and dignified personality and I do not consider that her work has been sufficiently appreciated.

Another group which visited Glasgow twice, and which I enjoyed, was called Braziliana. It was a mixed programme of dancing and mime, and they were truly natural and spontaneous dancers. They performed ballets on folk stories and dances, and included a great deal of improvisation. They had no formal technique, but this did not worry the audience because their enthusiasm was unbounded and infectious, and made up for any lack of skill and training. They literally would not stop dancing. After repeated calls when the final curtain came down, they still went on dancing, singing and shouting on a darkened stage until the staff forcibly removed them — and this was repeated every night.

Of the modern dance groups I have seen since I returned to London, the one that impressed me most was the Alvin Ailey Dancers. They were not a large group, and most of the members were Black; with a natural grace, and the men had wonderful physiques. There were a few white Caucasians, and when I saw their performance they danced no ballets to a story, but interpreted moods and situations; they used a variety of music, and the grouping and concerted movements were most interesting. This group did not show too obvious a ballet influence as many modern ones do.

Most classical ballet companies now include some modern work. The Ballet Rambert has now gone entirely modern: in the last performance I saw the dancers were clothed in tights, males and females were indistinguishable and there was not one skirt or flowing garment in the entire programme. However, some of the choreography was very good indeed, with interesting grouping and positioning of dancers.

Some companies I have seen appear to be terrified that the dancers should have the slightest relationship to each other either in grouping or movement. I have seen brilliant exhibitions of technique, but the dancers were spaced so far apart that they gave the impression of each doing individual practice, with dead-pan faces.

The last performance I attended was by a recently started school called the London School of Contemporary Dance, working, I believe, on the Martha Graham technique. There was variety in choreography and in costumes and very interesting lighting. I believe they are a young, dedicated and promising group.

I want to look back again, because modern developments in ballet owe a lot to the invasion by American musicals that hit London, and 'hit' is the right word, for the impact was terrific. They owed much of their success to the brilliant choreography of Agnes de Mille, for she was the first to use, in large-scale, popular productions, strong angular positions, and sudden jerky or heavy sustained movements, for dramatic effects in solo and group work, often intentionally tense and strained and mostly used for men. The obvious tough technique has now often been used in ballets and developed by male choreographers, Jerome Robbins, Michael Kidd and others. But it pleases me that it was all started by a woman — so I salute Agnes de Mille.

I believe it is of interest in relation to my attitude towards the classical ballet, that now that they have absorbed some of the modern idioms, I often find modern ballets produced by classical ballet companies of greater interest than those performed by the modern groups.

In the autumn of 1951, for the first time, a truly Scottish ballet was put on at Covent Garden by the Sadler's Wells Company (now the Royal Ballet). The ballet was called 'Donald of the Burthens', not an arresting title. The music was by Ian Whyte, then conductor of the Scottish BBC Orchestra; the choreography was by Massine, and the costumes and décor were by Colquhoun and MacBryde.

To my amazement I was commissioned by the BBC to review it on the Scottish Radio Art News. I learned later that I had only been asked because Marjorie Middleton, the principal ballet teacher in Edinburgh, was not available. However, I was delighted to go, and I rang up Ian Harrison, then editor of the *Scottish Field*, for which I had done sketches of the Sadler's Wells Ballet at the Edinburgh Festival, and asked if he would like me to do some sketches for him at Covent Garden. He accepted. I then asked the BBC If they could arrange for me to attend the dress rehearsals as well as the opening night. They said that it could easily be arranged and the theatre would be notified to expect me. When I arrived for the first rehearsal, a commissionaire from the front of the house was standing at the stage door, and as soon as I appeared, he said 'Excuse me Madam, but are you the lady from the BBC?'

He at once conducted me to the stalls, and presented me to Massine, Ninette de Valois and Marie Rambert, saying, "Excuse me, but this is the lady from the BBC.' I was received kindly and they all declared they knew my name and had heard of my Movement, which surprised me. I said I wanted to make sketches for the *Scottish Field* as well as to take notes for the broadcast, and asked if I could watch from the front of the circle as it provided a better view.

I found the ballet extremely interesting. I liked Ian Whyte's music very much, it was atmospheric and dramatic, and the way he introduced the pipes was fascinating. The piper played from the stage, standing well forward at the side, and it was Pipe Major Angus MacAulay, who had played in some of my ballets, but of course not with an orchestra. Having a piper actually playing with a full orchestra was a great innovation, but presented musical difficulties in the performance of the work

THE first performance of the Scottish ballet, "Donald of the Burthens," was given by the Sadler's Wells Ballet at Covent Garden recently. It seems strange that we are indebted to Massine and the Sadler's Wells Ballet for the first large-scale production of a Scottish Ballet, but actually the production was half-Scottish. The libretto and choreography were Massine's, but the music was by Ian Whyte, and costumes and decor by Robert Colquhoun and Robert MacBryde. Alexander Grant, as Donald, and the Sadler's Wells Company under the direction of Ninette de Valois, entered into the feeling of the Highland dance, and the ballet was well received bv a large first-night audience.

THE SKETCHES ON THIS PAGE WERE EXECUTED BY MARGARET MORRIS

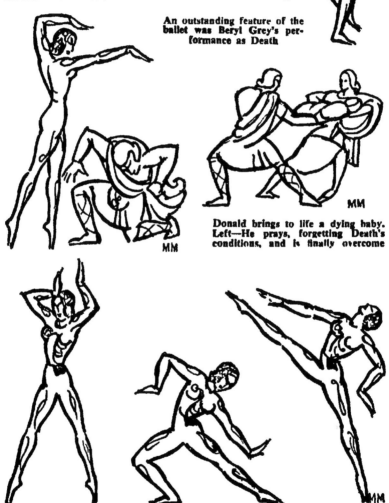

An outstanding feature of the ballet was Beryl Grey's performance as Death

Donald brings to life a dying baby. Left—He prays, forgetting Death's conditions, and is finally overcome

Poster advertising the ballet 'Donald of the Burthens' reproduced from the *Scottish Field*, February 1952.

which I feel was largely responsible for the fact that the ballet has never been repeated, though I believe parts of the music have been performed separately.

Massine's choreography was superb, and it was a wonderful example of how different techniques can be used to advantage. The corps de ballet were the people at the court of an early Celtic king, in plain straight garments, and the dances were simple with massed concerted movements and effective groupings. Alexander Grant as Donald the Highlander did the traditional dance steps while Beryl Grey, who played the part of Death, gave a most brilliant performance mainly on her points — and for once I found the point work entirely suitable, for she was the villain of the piece, dressed in scarlet tights with black markings. Again I salute Massine for the masterly way he used the point work, getting right away from the usual ballet technique, often using the knees bent and together, with no outward rotation. Beryl Grey looked wonderful, and the way she used her beautiful long legs with the added height on her points, gave a vicious poignancy to her movements, typifying evil.

I had been sent seats in the very centre of the stalls. During the interval I was looking round and saw hands waving over the side of the top gallery, and recognised several friends from the Glasgow press. When we met at the party after the show, and I told them how I came to be there, they said 'It is always the same — the BBC takes precedence everywhere!'

I had met Beryl Grey during the rehearsals, and made sketches in her dressing-room. I liked her very much, particularly for her wide range of interests. I told her of my ambition to found a really Scottish Ballet, and she urged me to go forward with it. Some years later, when the scheme for the Scottish National Ballet was under way, and when many people were trying to persuade me to include classical ballet, I wrote to Beryl Grey and asked her to tell me what she felt about it. She answered at once, and gave me permission to use her letter on our appeal circular. I will quote from it here:

'I am very happy that you are making this bid to form a company again . . . After thinking it over, I really feel that you are wise not to include classical ballet, but to concentrate on the style of dancing which is unique to Scotland and natural to them . . . I am sure that the strength of the company, as you so rightly say, is in its source of Scottish legend, folklore, etc . . . I would like to wish you every success in this venture and please, if there is anything I can do to help, do let me know. I feel sure you have something to offer the world in this field so good luck.'

This letter remains a pleasant memory. To find sympathy and understanding in a star from the opposing school of dancing was an inspiration at a most difficult time.

During my twenty-one years in Glasgow, I have been on radio and television several times. I recorded my life for the Woman's Hour. *My Galsworthy Story*, which I wrote for the centenary, aroused a great deal of interest, and I was asked to attend the dress rehearsal of his play *Justice* in order to discuss it on Late Night Line-up after the opening. I was reminded of my Covent Garden experience, for when I arrived at the St Martin's Theatre, I received the same treatment. I doubt if I shall ever feel as important as I do when I am 'the lady from the BBC'.

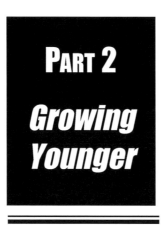

PART 2

Growing Younger

Through Diet, Exercise and Mental Attitude

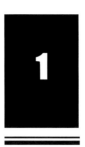

1

Am I an Exception?

THE ANSWER IS NO. We all have the same body mechanisms and digestive processes, so that even allowing for individual tendencies and allergies, the same basic health rules apply to everyone. I am giving my personal experiences, and the conclusions I have reached over a long period of trial and error, in the hope that they may prove of some help to some people.

I admit I have been blessed with a sound constitution and my personal life has been extraordinarily happy. But ever since I was sixteen I have been consistently overworked, and I have never been free of financial and other worries connected with the running of schools, producing ballets and putting on theatre shows, always with inadequate finances. Many times I have driven myself almost to breaking point, and have only managed to carry on through short fasts and strict attention to diet.

Why I Don't Eat Meat

I am often asked why I do not eat meat or animal products, whether on grounds of health, or for sentimental reasons? The answer is both. Even as a child I was devoted to animals, and it seemed to me entirely illogical, if you loved them, to eat them. Much later I became convinced of the importance of avoiding flesh foods for health. Several times during my life, for convenience, I have returned to an ordinary diet, but each time the rapid deterioration in health and vitality was so obvious that since 1930 I have not touched meat, fish or fowl. I have also

169

avoided sugar and starchy foods, eating almost exclusively fresh fruits and green vegetables: and I can honestly say that I am practically never tired, never catch colds or 'flu, and have more energy than I had forty years ago.

To the Over-Forties

I am sure that everyone over forty — male and female — would like to grow younger instead of older. I maintain this can be done. If it sounds a fantastic statement, the explanation is simply that most people age prematurely, through bad eating and drinking, lack of exercise, and a wrong mental attitude to life, and that, by changing bad habits to good, in a great many cases lost youth can be regained.

Nowadays there are so many books on diet and exercise, and on cults of various kinds, I doubt if there has ever been a time when people were so health-conscious. Then why all this premature aging? Certainly the expectation of life is longer than it has ever been in the civilised world, but this seems to me a very doubtful benefit. Are the majority much healthier or happier? Does not medical science often keep people alive who would be better dead?

If you think I am exaggerating, look around at your friends between forty and sixty. How few of the women retain a youthful figure and a joy in life. How many of the men are either paunchy or flabby, and lacking in vitality and virility? These are only the outward signs of degeneration. How often do you hear complaints of fatigue, recurring headaches, rheumatic pains, or regrets at loss of energy and youthful vigour? And how many people whom you have thought of as healthy develop some latent disease, have operations and nervous breakdowns or even suddenly die?

Most disorders are simply the result of years of wrong living, and therefore, if deterioration has not gone too far, it is possible to do something about it. Obviously there are contagious diseases, hereditary tendencies, allergies and so on, where medical advice should be sought. It is advisable, particularly for older people, to consult a qualified doctor before making any drastic changes, but it should be one in sympathy with progressive ideas on fasting, diet and exercise. Though Basic Breathing and other simple exercises can be done with benefit at any age, and immediately following operations and childbirth, there are some conditions — which may be unsuspected — where movement is contra-indicated, or where changes in diet might be dangerous. It may take some time to obtain results, because all changes involving the whole organism must be made gradually.

I am talking to men as much as to women, because in structure and physiology, except for the sex organs, they are alike. All the other systems of the body — for example the respiratory system and the alimentary canal — are similar, and whether you are male or female, for health and happiness, there must be a balanced harmony of mind and body. Once the realisation has come to you that you could look better and feel younger, then the question is how?

Combining the Three Essentials

I believe the secret of success in growing younger is always to combine the three essentials, diet, exercise and mental attitude. I think the big mistake that is usually made is to concentrate on one aspect only. One book tells you that everything can be controlled through the mind, or through spiritual beliefs: another that fasting and diet are all that is necessary: and of course I should say that you only need to do my exercises to acquire eternal youth! But I cannot honestly say this, though in the past year I have personally rediscovered my method by practising it again, and I am glad to say that I find my exercises are even better than I thought. I must state emphatically that to re-establish health and vigour, correct diet is even more important than exercise, and therefore I put it first.

Many people will say that mental attitude should come first, so I give a diagram, on the next page, which I hope makes my point of view clear. As I have said, all three must be integrated, but the emphasis may for a time be more on one side than another.

I visualise a pyramid with mental attitude at the apex — the dominating factor: but in building a pyramid you must begin at the base, and therefore diet and exercise, though eventually of lesser importance, must be the foundation on which you build. The reason for this is that if the body is encumbered by poisonous matter from years of wrong living, clogging the liver and other organs and the whole of the digestive tract, clear thinking becomes impossible, and the so-called spiritual powers are inevitably impaired. This happens to the majority of people as they grow older.

To those who believe that all can be achieved through the spirit, I would say that no matter what we believe, while we are on this earth we can only function and convey through our bodies. Therefore, whatever our beliefs, ambitions and aspirations, we should keep our bodies as youthful and efficient as possible, and learn how to grow old happily and gracefully.

The thing to remember is that the longer you may have to live, the more important it is to feel well and enjoy life. I am not afraid of dying — but I am very much afraid I may have to live a long time!

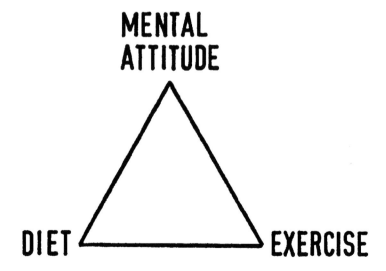

MENTAL
ATTITUDE

DIET   EXERCISE

2

Diet

I SHOULD FIRST LIKE TO STATE EMPHATICALLY that enjoyment of what you eat and drink is essential to health. But you must be able to distinguish between enjoyment and craving. The enjoyment of right foods is the result of healthy hunger, but an irresistible craving for things like tea, coffee, sweets, rich and highly seasoned foods, curries etc, shows that the body has been more or less poisoned by these particular foods, which create a craving similar to that produced by tobacco, alcohol and drugs, only in a less deadly degree. The results take longer to become evident, and this is also a danger, for you can poison yourself quite respectably on tea or coffee all your life, and no one will try to stop you.

It is one of the great fallacies to believe that your body knows what it needs. If it is in perfect health it does. Healthy children love raw carrots, apples etc, and — if they have never been given them — feel no desire for cakes and sweets which cause tooth decay and undermine health. But how many people over forty enjoy the perfect health indicated by freedom from cravings or dependence on stimulants?

Any craving indicates some bodily deficiency or maladjust-ment, and it is the job of one's medical adviser to find the cause and the remedy. But few will admit that more often than not the cause is a lifetime of wrong feeding, eating destructive instead of constructive foods. Of course we all need sugar, children especially, but it should be natural sugar, such as is found in molasses, honey, and fresh and dried fruits.

I am convinced that the prevalent ill-health of all the civilised nations is due to a great extent to malnutrition: more people suffer from under-nourishment through over-eating than from not having enough to eat. This is because it is not the quantity eaten, but the amount the body can assimilate that nourishes it, and gives health and energy.

It has been said that of the average mixed diet of so-called good foods not more than one-sixth of the intake is assimilated. The rest clogs the intestines and has to be disposed of. A certain amount of bulk and roughage is of course necessary, but when what is eaten consists mainly of rich fatty foods and starches, digestive troubles occur, causing liver upsets, headaches and fatigue. This is because all the waste products are not being eliminated, but held up in some part of the intestine, where they produce that most common of all complaints, constipation, to which so much poor health and many diseases can be directly traced. I believe that the majority of people in Britain today are constipated but don't know it, because most people think that constipation occurs only in the lower bowel — the colon — and that they are all right if it acts once a day, however inadequately.

Erhert's Theories

At this point, I want to speak of a little-known German dietician named Erhert, because his theories have helped me more than any others I have come across. Most of the medical profession who have heard of him consider him eccentric: but a few consider that his ideas, though perhaps too extreme, should be investigated. It was one of these, Dr Pink of the Stonefield Maternity Home, who in 1930 gave me a copy of Erhert's book *Mucusless Diet Healing System*. Erhert's special theory was that the accumulation of mucus in the body was the basic cause of all disease, because, he claimed, if the body were not clogged with mucus it could even resist infection. He believed that the right and natural diet for all human beings was one of fruits, nuts and green-leaf vegetables. All other foods, he held, formed mucus in varying degrees, but he advised a careful transition diet, allowing root vegetables, wholemeal bread and even yoghurt and cheeses to begin with. For years he had a clinic where he claimed he cured hundreds of patients, many of whom had been given up as hopeless. The cure consisted of very carefully controlled fasts, interspersed with special diets.

Erhert himself went in for spectacular fasts. For over four weeks at a time he was shut up in a kind of glass case where, continually watched, he took nothing but water, and at the end claimed he had more energy than before, doing strenuous exercises and taking long walks. This was to prove his theory that if the body were really clean and free from mucus, it could derive energy almost indefinitely from water and air alone.

I have recounted this in the hope that it may make some impression on those people who think they will die if they miss so much as one meal. I do not advocate long fasts, nor indeed did Erhert, who always stressed their danger unless the body was really internally clean. If it is not, the accumulated poisons pass into the bloodstream and may cause death: but he insists that even in death from starvation, this is caused by the poisons, not by the mere lack of food.

I am ashamed to say I have never had the time — nor the courage — to try a fast of more than four days: but I can state from long personal experience that a cold can be cured in two days, if you stop eating as soon as you are aware of it, take only hot or cold liquids, and don't eat even fruit, and never biscuits or toast. All sweet drinks should be avoided. A hot toddy at night, however, with lemon, honey and even a little whisky, is quite good. The purists on health cures won't agree with me on this — which reminds me of a true story. One morning in Paris I was walking past the Café du Dôme in Montparnasse, when a woman artist I knew waved to me, grinning broadly. I remarked that she looked very well. 'Oh yes,' she said, 'but I've been very ill, and the doctor made me fast for four days and have nothing but liquids. Now I'm feeling on top of the world!'. There was a large Pernod by her side. Evidently it had never occurred to her that alcohol might not be included in the cure.

What to Drink

The whole question of alcohol is very controversial, most vegetarians and nature-cure people being entirely against it. Meat eaters expect vegetarians to be kill-joys, and are always amazed when I accept wine. Perhaps because I — and my family before me — have lived so much in France, wine drinking seems natural to me. Wine is a product of the grape, with no cruelty involved in its manufacture, and it is a very pleasant and fairly harmless stimulant, if not taken in excess.

Undeniably, pure fresh water — from a crystal spring — is the ideal health drink, but not many of us can obtain this. Most drinking water is now rendered harmless, even abroad, but I wonder at what expense to its revitalising qualities? Yet even so it seems that almost any water is better than none, though it should be drunk between, not with, meals. I only drink plain water last thing at night, during the night if I wake, and first thing in the morning. I am never thirsty, and do not drink at meals except when tempted with special wines.

Unfermented grape juice is probably better than wine for the health, and it tastes good too, but there is no kick to it! Of course if you are in really perfect health, there is no need for any kick, but for most of us, even if we live on pure foods, the stress and strain of modern life require a mild stimulant. There is not much joy in life nowadays, and I believe that all simple pleasures not actually detrimental to health should be encouraged.

The cocktail habit, however, is undoubtedly bad, the mixed strong alcohols being very destructive to the delicate membranes of the stomach and intestines. A mild *aperitif*, a glass of sherry, or a small whisky and water, are relatively harmless and do stimulate appetite, but I doubt the wisdom of letting even these become a habit. Personally I like a well-warmed burgundy as a pre-dinner drink.

Besides liking wine, I am even more enthusiastic about fresh grapes when they are really good. Many varieties have no taste at all, but when those that are full of flavour are available, I often make a meal of grapes alone. So, although I do drink wine, I do not agree with the man who, when his hostess pressed him to try some specially beautiful grapes, replied: 'Thank you, madam, but I do not like the juice of the grape in capsules!'

Wine Versus Tea or Coffee

I am rather sad to think that only a few vegetarians will agree with me that wine is a more natural and less harmful drink than either tea or coffee, for these I consider should be listed as dangerous drugs. Coffee is a strong heart stimulant and can be useful as such, but many people take it four times a day and cannot do without it. Tea, on the other hand, is a less powerful stimulant, but it is far worse for the digestion than coffee, especially for meat-eaters, because of the tannin it contains. The traditional high tea, with meat, starch, sweets and strong tea, is about the worst possible dietetic combination.

In my opinion, both tea and coffee should count as drugs, as both create an almost irresistible craving. I know, because for years I was a tea addict. As I only drank weak China tea, I imagined it was harmless, not realising that, as I drank five or six cups at a time, it added up to one strong cup — and this I took five or six times a day. In time I noticed that I craved for it more and more. Whenever I was tired or worried, I would make a large pot of China tea. When I noticed also that I was becoming nervous and that my digestion was impaired, I realised that I must stop my tea-drinking habits. I began drinking Matte tea instead, and as this does not create any craving I drank far less, and soon improved in health. However, it was twenty years before I lost my craving for tea completely.

It distresses me that so many vegetarians are tea addicts, and that they also poison themselves with starch and sweets into the bargain. The only thing against the drinking of wine is the price. Tea, and even coffee, are certainly cheaper. And here I must give a warning about the cheapest wines: while these can be safely drunk where they are grown and made, some will not travel, so vin ordinaire in Paris or London is sometimes reinforced with cheap alcohol, which may be positively harmful.

White wines are on the whole more acid than red. French doctors often warn their patients to avoid white and rosé, although this may not apply to first-class wines. There are many cheap red wines from various countries that do not seem acid, and I believe that a little red wine can be beneficial, whereas tea or coffee can only be harmful. Spirits too can be dangerous, and I do not believe they should be taken regularly.

As to the question of diet, I suggest keeping an open mind and not just accepting what conventional dieticians advocate. Often the so-called cranks are genuine pioneers who are eventually proved right. I am only restating what several have said before when I maintain that only living foods give life and energy. Fresh fruits, green salads, raw vegetables and freshly ground wheat, are still alive — while cooked vegetables, and wholemeal bread for example are not. Admittedly these last have their uses, but are they really necessary? Erhert thinks not.

Animals Eat Living Foods

In support of the living food theory, all vegetarian animals in their natural state eat only living foods — grass, roots, nuts, grains and fruits. Carnivorous animals eat their food freshly killed and raw. Meat eaters take note: to extract any goodness out of meat, you should eat it raw. By the time it reaches you it has probably been frozen and then cooked — many meat dishes are even cooked twice — so that all you derive from them is uric acid and other harmful products.

An idea that many people seem to have is that you must eat muscle in order to make muscle. This is really too fantastic. Look at the elephants and buffaloes — where do they get their tremendous muscles? And horses, especially race horses? Think of the strength, energy and endurance which they derive from living grains. This brings me to the point that even compost-grown wholemeal, when made into bread and cooked, is merely second-hand nourishment. Only so long as the grain is unbroken does it retain the germ of life; if planted in suitable soil or put in water, it will create new life by sprouting. If, instead of eating bread, you eat a small quantity of freshly ground wheat, moistened with fruit juice or milk, you are eating living food, capable of giving you new life. There is nothing new in this idea. When I was seventeen my mother used to buy Christian's Unfired Bread, consisting of raw crushed wheat pressed into a kind of biscuit: but it was very dry and dull, and the wheat, having been crushed, must already have lost much of its life.

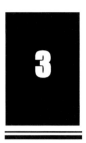

3

What I Eat

I AM SO OFTEN ASKED WHAT I EAT that I will make a list for those who are interested.

On waking (any time between 5am and 8am). The juice of a lemon, freshly cut, and a good spoonful of molasses in warm water.

Soon after: a large pot of Matte tea with a little honey. (After this I usually work for an hour or two and then take my bath).

Breakfast: one more cup of Matte tea, wholemeal bread with sweet almond cream or honey. (I omit this if I sleep late.)

Mid-morning: lemon and molasses again — very stimulating.

Lunch (any time between 11.30 and 1pm). Fresh fruit, grated apples with orange or pineapple juice, sometimes melon or grapefruit. A large lettuce salad, with a dressing of the best olive oil and fresh lemon juice, a very little salt and black freshly ground pepper. Colman's mustard can be added, and chopped onion or garlic. I eat this basic salad each day, varying it by adding celery, cucumber, red peppers, grated carrot or raw beetroot, endive, or any cooked vegetable left over from the night before. Tomatoes can be added every day, but if just cut and thrown in, they make the lettuce go limp from too much moisture. My method with tomatoes is to put them in boiling water, count seven, skin them, cut them in half and then scoop out the juice before putting them in my salad. Raisins, dates and nuts can also be added, and even tinned vegetables and fruits if you crave more variety. The new combinations that can be made are almost endless.

180

Tea: Matte tea again if at home, very weak Russian tea or fruit juice if not. Nothing to eat.

Dinner (not less than six hours after lunch). Any vegetables, but mostly green ones, including spring cabbage, spinach and sprouts, cooked in a casserole or boiled, in which case I save the water for soup next day. I use various herbs to flavour the vegetables, and I eat them with a dressing of olive oil and lemon. If I have visitors, I use butter for those who prefer it.

My soups are of the French peasant variety, with vegetables cut large. I use lots of onions, and sometimes garlic, and mashed potatoes for thickening, often with two or three different herbs. Basil is my favourite, and then tarragon. My friends are always enthusiastic and ask for my recipe: but I cook by inspiration and tasting, throwing in anything that is handy and that will add to the flavour, even tinned beans or spaghetti in tomato on occasion.

I sometimes make omelettes, the French kind my mother taught me to make when I was a child. She also taught me to make pastry, but I stopped making it long ago, because the combination of grease and starch is, as a friend of mine put it, 'dietetically disastrous'!

I serve cheese and biscuits, and coffee if desired. I don't poison myself, but if it makes them happy I poison my friends.

I adore garlic, and it is a wonderful internal disinfectant. It must be admitted, however, that the aroma is apt to cling for days, which may interfere with your social and amorous life. Dr Rollier of Leysin made his patients eat it every day, and he maintained that, eaten with chopped parsley, it left no recurring smell. I do this, but am not fully convinced.

Eating Out

Eating out is no longer the problem it was for vegetarians fifty years ago. Now every restaurant has salads, egg and cheese dishes, melons, grapefruits, and often globe artichokes and avocados. Even pubs nowadays are beginning to serve salad lunches.

How to Start

If you find that you are growing tired more quickly than you used to, that you no longer have your former drive and energy, and that life has lost much of its interest for you, try doing without the occasional meal. The evening meal is best, because you will miss it least, and if you take a hot drink on going to bed you should be able to sleep. It is advisable to take a laxative before and after even a short fast, the object of the fast being to draw out the latent poisons in your system, and this is apt to make you feel miserable: but the worse you feel the more it shows how badly your body was in need of a purge.

There are several 'nature treatment' homes (if you can afford them) where this is done for you, efficiently but drastically because most people insist on quick results. Home treatments take much longer, but if kept up they yield more lasting results.

A Short Fast

A 24-hour fast is far more effective than missing one meal only, and it is easy if, instead of starting in the early morning when you have to face the whole day without a meal you begin your fast after midday lunch one day and finish before a 1 o'clock lunch the following day. In this way you eat your midday meal on both days, yet you have given your digestive system a clear 24-hour rest. On each day, lunch should consist of fruit and green salad only.

It should be remembered that as one grows older all the processes of the body tend to slow down, and food takes longer to pass through the intestines. Usually, people take less exercise and consume more rich food and drink as they grow older. If food is taken too often, the previous meal has not passed as far down the intestine as it should, and the next meal causes digestive disturbances.

Many people claim to have headaches or to feel sick if they eat nothing between meals. The explanation is that when the stomach is really empty, the process of elimination begins, and if the body is clogged with half-digested foods and the resulting mucus and poisons, some of these reach the bloodstream and cause headaches and other ailments. As soon as food is taken again the process of elimination is arrested, and therefore the body is temporarily relieved of discomfort. But the addition of new food, when the old is already causing trouble, does nothing to remove the cause of that trouble.

So if going without a meal, or fasting for 24 hours, makes you feel really wretched, you should seek medical advice on natural progressive lines.

Night Starvation

There is no such thing as night starvation. It is in fact night poisoning, due to the causes I have already explained. Inability to sleep, or constant waking during the night, unless directly attributable to acute worry or emotional disturbance, is nearly always due to wrong eating or drinking, or to eating too much, or too late, of even the right foods. Too much alcohol is also apt to over-stimulate. Acidity, fermentation and other processes can all disturb sleep, even though there may be no obvious digestive discomfort.

It is true that a light snack will often make sleep possible, but it should not become a habit. Rather, heed the warning that difficulty in sleeping is a sign that you are not in good condition. A really clean body has no difficulty in sleeping. I sleep wonderfully well, except on occasions of acute anxiety. But I have found that after a day or two on liquids only, when I feel really empty, I sleep longer and better than ever. I take a warm lemon drink before retiring, and this is both helpful and comforting. It should be remembered, however, that milk curdles and becomes a food inside you, so all milk drinks should be avoided.

Humour Yourself

All habits are acquired; so all habits can be changed, but only if the desire to change is stronger than the desire to continue.

Only a very few people have the strength of character to decide one day that some habit — such as smoking — must stop, and live up to their decision.

Use stimulants if you must, but with full consciousness of the dangers involved. Eat the wrong foods occasionally, but try not to do so too often. Even drink too much on occasion. It will not do you as much harm as regular wrong eating, or drinking with meals. Above all, be honest with yourself. I mean this very seriously. A quotation from *Hamlet* comes into my mind. (I used to know by heart all the Shakespeare plays I acted in as a child.) Polonius says to Laertes: 'To thine own self be true, and then 'twill follow, as the night the day, thou canst not then be false to any man.'

Transition Diet

Begin by cutting down or omitting, the things that are generally admitted to be bad for you, including all fried foods, all rich and heavy sauces and gravies, white bread, white sugar, sweets, pastries and all sweet biscuits, fatty meats, butter and eggs and anything else that is heavy in animal fats.

Try not to have more than two courses at each meal, but eat as much as you want of your main course.

Decide always to eat a large green salad at one meal, and plenty of green vegetables at another, even though you add some meat or fish at each.

Eat fresh fruit by itself, not at the end of a meal; at mid-morning, for instance, or in the evening instead of tea or coffee with biscuits. Or begin each meal with fruit.

One of Erhert's ideas is to plan a meal of several courses in this order: fresh fruits, followed by green salad, then cooked vegetables, and finally egg, cheese or even meat dishes. (You will eat less of these at the end than at the beginning of the meal).

One last word of warning. Do not suddenly change to an all fruit diet. You will most probably regret it.

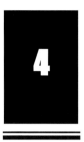

Restarting Exercise

WHATEVER YOUR AGE, you can always grow younger: younger, that is, than you feel and look at that particular time. When the realisation comes to you that youth depends on health of body and mind, you already have the right mental attitude. Everything now seems to be fiercely competitive, whether in the business, professional or social sectors. Perhaps it always was so, but the pace of life has certainly increased, and everything is now on an international scale. Another big difference is that the emphasis now is on youth. So the over-forties, men as well as women, need to arrest oncoming age and renew their energy by reforming their diet and doing some kind of concentrated exercise.

But first it is important to know what you are aiming for. What are the essentials upon which the proper functioning of the body depends? Obviously not the movements of the arms and legs — although these assist the circulation — because all the vital organs are in the trunk. Many years ago a book was written by Dr F. A. Hornibrook called *The Culture of the Abdomen*.[8] It was entirely sound in theory, and it pointed the way towards an appreciation of the value of exercising.

Lack of time and of inclination often prevent people from doing exercises. This has led me to devise exercises involving the most essential movements only. I have spread them over the whole day, on the principle of doing a little often. I shall describe these later, with diagrams.

Importance of Correct Breathing

I should like to place particular emphasis on breathing, since it is the most vital function of the body. It is the first sign of life, and the cessation of breathing is death.

Most people are terrified of going without food, but they live, and often sleep, without fresh air, and are not at all worried about the lack of oxygen. Yet oxygen is the one absolute essential to life. As Erhert and others have proved, life can continue for weeks without any food at all, for days even without water, but only for a few seconds without oxygen. How many people bother to learn how to breathe so as to fill and empty their lungs adequately? Yet this is the best safeguard against infections that enter through the respiratory tract. Oxygen is connected with the combustion of fats in the body, which means that deep breathing assists those attempting to reduce their weight.

Spinal Mobility

Next in importance I put the mobilising of the spine, because the nerves leading to all the organs of the body radiate from each side of the spine. As the body grows older the spine becomes shorter, because the discs between the vertebrae tend to shrink, which may cause pressure on the nerves and interfere with the functioning of the organs they supply.

If the spine is kept mobile, retaining its full range of movement, the circulation is improved, and if the lateral movements of which the spine is capable are included in any exercises, the small intrinsic muscles of the spine will retain their tone and elasticity. It is the atrophy of these muscles that allows the discs, when a sudden movement occurs, to slip out of position.

Posture

The spine is most obviously connected with posture, keeping the body upright. I will deal with the correction of faulty postures later when I describe the exercises: but here I want to stress that, as one grows older, it is necessary to make a conscious effort to keep a really upright position, because of the pull of gravity. In both extreme youth and in age, a definite effort must be made. Young children struggle to stand upright, fall down, and at last manage to keep erect.

The digestive system is your lifeline, and the abdomen is vital in relation to exercise, because it is the only part that can be directly affected by pressure and twisting movements. In this connection Basic Breathing is the most important of all, and that is why I integrate it in all the exercises.

Stretching and Relaxing

The alternate stretching and relaxing of the tendons of the body, and the alternating of muscular contraction and relaxation, are of the utmost importance for the circulation of the blood. It should be remembered that, because of the downward pull of gravity, it is especially the extensor muscles of the back and neck that the over-forties need to strengthen.

Opposition Movements

In all human movement, the most fundamental law is that of the opposition working of the arms and legs. As in walking, running, hurdling, bowling, tennis, football and other activities when any effort is made, the balance of the body must be kept by a set of muscles working in opposition. This fundamental law is overlooked in most gymnastic exercises.

The positions collected from Greek vases by Raymond Duncan, which I call Basic Held Positions, are perfect examples of this law of opposition in a form that can be practised so as to strengthen the necessary muscles. Athletes who have consulted me have found them invaluable. I do not include them in my Daily Routines as it is difficult to perform them correctly without instruction; but the principle of opposition can be used even when exercising on a chair. I shall explain later how this can be done.

Walking

I consider walking a much overrated exercise, particularly when done by the middle-aged, with a bag or a briefcase tucked under one arm. If both arms can swing freely, and Basic Breathing is synchronised with the walking, then it is beneficial. Even so, five minutes' concentrated exercise would be much better for you.

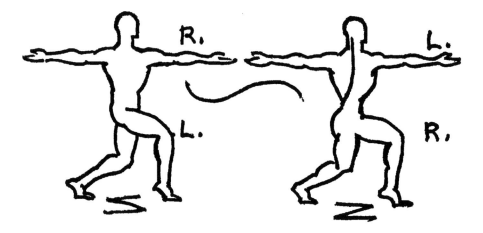

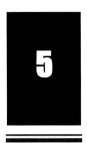

THE RIGHT MENTAL ATTITUDE IS ESSENTIAL to happiness. I have not studied psychology, although I have a great respect for this branch of medicine, but I find it is often used as an excuse for not changing bad habits. With regard to psychoanalysis, I try to keep an open mind, but I am convinced that if more people corrected their bad eating and drinking habits, there would be less for the psychoanalysts to do.

A lot is written about thought transference, hypnosis and auto-suggestion. It seems to me that all the new schools of thought, religious and philosophical, are based largely on rediscoveries of old wisdom. More than half a century ago, the French scientist Coué rediscovered for the then modern world the power of auto-suggestion and demonstrated on hundreds of patients that many physical, as well as mental illnesses could be cured merely by repeating a silly sounding doggerel which automatically applied itself to every ailment. I remember there were jokes about it at the time — Fleur quotes the words in John Galsworthy's *The Forsyte Saga*, for example — but it had to be admitted that, amazing as it seemed, in a large proportion of cases, it worked. The formula ran:

Every day and in every way
I am getting better and better.

Or in the original French:

*Tous les jours et à tout point de vue
Je vais de mieux en mieux*

The moral of this is that it is the *idea* that matters — that the subconscious, which successfully controls the functioning of our extremely complex bodies, can be directed, by commands from the conscious, to give special attention to putting right anything that has gone wrong.

Coué was insistent that this was not a matter of faith, and that faith healing was merely the operating of this scientific law. He maintained that it was not necessary to believe that you could be cured. If you repeated the formula often enough, you would be cured despite your lack of conviction. For several years there was discussion about this, but after Coué's, death interest lapsed, although I am sure his ideas have been used in other forms.

Ever since I first heard of Coué, I believed that his idea should be linked in some way with my work, but I could not then see how this might be done. It has only been during the last ten years, while I have been evolving my personal routines, that I realised I could do them to Coué's formula, with some adaptations. So I have given the words with the exercises, as I have used them for several years now with great success.

Before beginning your exercises, decide exactly what you want to achieve. Try and relax and not set up any opposition within yourself. Tell yourself that what you want to do will be easy. Cultivate patience. Observe everything around you. Analyse your reasons for being attached to tobacco, alcohol, rich foods or sweets, and if you can relax and not worry, suddenly the way may be clear to a change in your habits.

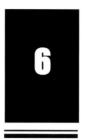

BEFORE DESCRIBING THE DAILY ROUTINES, I should like to give a clear explanation of two main factors, breathing and spinal mobility. I have already said something about the importance of breathing. Now I am giving an outline of the anatomy of the parts concerned, as well as the mechanism of Basic Breathing and how it can best be learnt. This should be thoroughly understood and practised alone first, so that it will be done instinctively with all the Daily Routines. If the breathing is incorrectly done, at least half the value of the exercise will be lost.

Anatomy of Breathing

The lungs are situated, together with the heart, in the upper part of the body, the thorax. They are separated from all the other organs by a sheet of muscle, the diaphragm, which stretches from the front of the body to the back, very like the floor of a house. Through this floor pass various tubes: the trachea for air, the oesophagus for food and the largest blood vessels in the body. The diaphragm is elastic and intimately concerned with breathing.

Points to Remember

The apices of the lungs come up into the neck, behind and above the collar-bones or clavicles, and it is very important to draw the air right up into the apices.

On full inspiration, as the lower part of the lungs expands, the diaphragm descents, and on expiration, as the lungs are emptied, it rises again.

The pulling in of the abdomen on expiration (as done in Basic Breathing) exerts an inward and upward pressure on the intestines.

This, alternating with the downward pressure of the diaphragm on inspiration, gives a kind of auto massage to the intestines, most beneficial to the digestion and helpful in combating any tendency to stasis (constipation).

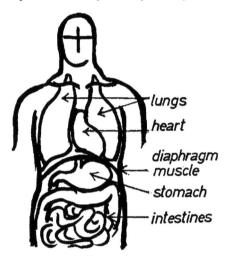

ANATOMY OF BREATHING

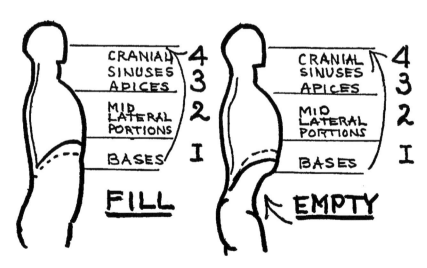

BASIC BREATHING

Basic Breathing: The Mechanism

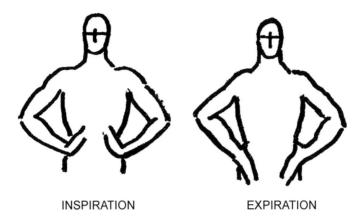

INSPIRATION   EXPIRATION

Inspiration

No conscious muscular contraction. Expand the lungs fully from the base upwards, endeavouring to draw the air up into the cranial sinuses. The mouth must be kept closed, and air should be drawn in through the nose.

Expiration

Contract and draw up the lower abdomen, keeping the contraction throughout the whole expiration. Let the air come out through the lips gently, with a soft whistling sound. Allow the chest wall to relax at the end of the expiration. The easiest way to learn Basic Breathing is lying on your back, then sitting on a chair, then standing and finally while walking. The number of steps you hold each breath for will depend on your lung capacity. If you learn this form of breathing, you will derive great benefit.

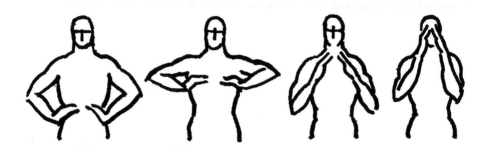

BASIC BREATHING: STANDING

To begin with, it is helpful if you indicate with your fingers which part of the lungs is extended. But once the method has been thoroughly learned and understood, this is no longer necessary. Basic Breathing can be practised either sitting or standing, in the following way.

Place hands on hips, with *thumbs behind* at waistline, where they remain throughout, being used as a pivot.

It is sometimes objected that it is not natural to breathe out through the mouth. But this is an exercise, and more air can be expelled through the mouth than through the nose.

In repose, or when breathing to induce sleep, the mouth should be kept shut, the air entering and leaving by the nose. But in exertion it is a very different matter. Just try expelling the air *quickly* through the nose! And is it unnatural for air to leave the body through the mouth while talking?

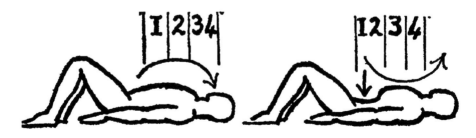

BASIC BREATHING: LYING

Anatomy of the Spine

Everyone should know what are the normal curves of the spine in relation to good posture, and also what are the most common defects that occur as the body begins to age. I shall explain the full range of movement of which the normal spine is capable. Most people are unaware of the amount of mobility which is possible, and which I maintain is of the utmost importance to health.

There are four physiological curves in the spine, which are developed as an infant begins to move its body and lift its head. It is perhaps not generally known that a baby is born with a flat back and flat feet. It is as the muscles grow, through constant movement and effort, that the curves of the spine and the arches of the feet develop. Any exaggeration of the natural curves becomes pathological.

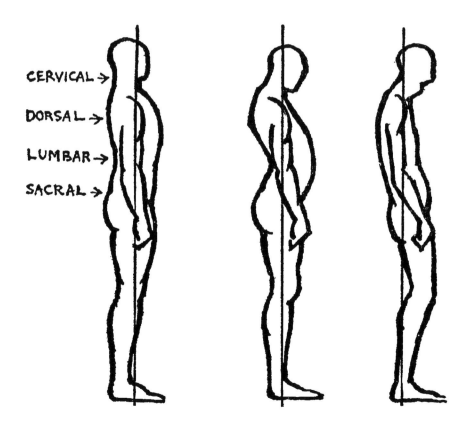

CERVICAL →

DORSAL →

LUMBAR →

SACRAL →

I am not dealing here with remedial exercises, but so few spines have perfectly normal curves that I am giving a few useful corrective positions in which to practise Basic Breathing. With ageing, round shoulders and round backs are by far the most common defects, due partly, as I have said, to the downward pull of gravity. If associated with hollow or flat back, the positions below may be used.

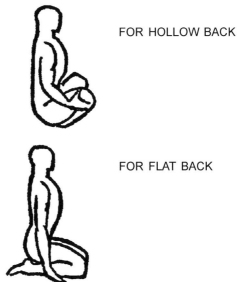

FOR HOLLOW BACK

FOR FLAT BACK

'Ironing out your spine', described later, is the most useful exercise for halting middle-aged stoop, or round backs. Any lateral curvature (scoliosis) usually first noticed through one shoulder being lower than the other should be reported at once to your doctor. I have treated many people with this defect, but only under medical instructions.

Anatomically, the spine is only capable of four movements (see page 197). But it is also capable of a fifth movement, a lateral movement obtained by a double side flexion performed simultaneously. A well known example is the Indian dancer's lateral movement of the head, which is achieved by a *right* side flexion of the cervical spine combined with a *left* side flexion of the sub-occipital joint; or, for a movement towards the other side, a *left* side flexion of the cervical spine combined with a right flexion of the sub-occipital joint. I have found that similar

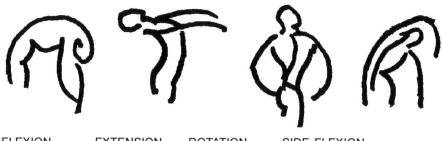

FLEXION   EXTENSION   ROTATION   SIDE FLEXION

movements were possible also in the lumbar region, involving the lower dorsal region.

All movements of the spine in the dorsal and lumbar regions can be done in two ways, by moving the pelvis or by fixing the pelvis and moving the thorax.

This lateral movement occurs in Spanish, Indian and other native dances involving circular movements of the pelvis, but I do not think it has been isolated and used as in my pelvic and thoracic mobility exercises.

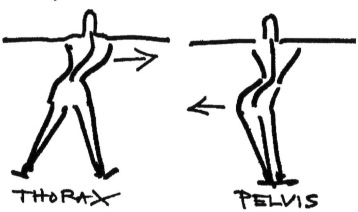

THORAX   PELVIS

About the Diagrams on pages 201 onwards

These stick figures I have drawn look stiff and angular, whereas the movements they depict should be flowing and easy, though accurate. The sexlessness of the figures makes them uninteresting, but they are obviously highly suitable in depicting exercises intended for men as well as for women, since each can follow them with equal ease.

I have used some of the signs from my own notation to indicate the way in which the transition from one position to another should be made. A plain line indicates a sweeping gesture, a wavy line indicates relaxation, or a relaxed bend and stretch from one position to the next.

Imitate the figures as if you were looking at yourself in a mirror, right and left being reversed. Where necessary, the letters R and L are used. The arrows indicate the direction of a movement.

Bars and Rhythm

As all the exercises can be done to music, bars, time signatures and repeat signs have been used as in musical notation.

The beats in each bar are written above the figures; the beat on which a position is reached is underlined, as it is not always possible to put the figure exactly under the correct beat because of lack of space. For example, in the fourth bar of Breathe and Contract (see p209) the position adopted on the first beat is held for the remaining three beats.

The breathing throughout must be Basic Breathing, which means that the lower abdomen should be drawn in firmly on each outward breath, though this is not stated each time.

Using Coué's Words

It is best to think the words, while keeping the rhythm of the exercise, for though the words can be fitted to the four beats in the bar, if they are spoken aloud the breathing may be impeded. It is of course quite possible to contract the abdomen while speaking and indeed this is often done by singers and speakers.

Daily Routines

The following is a list of exercises to be done each day:

In bed: 'Stretch to wake'	1 minute
On getting up: 'Energising exercise'	5 minutes
In transit: 'Invisible exercise'	~~2 minutes~~
At the office: 'Renewing exercise'	2 minutes
At home: 'Armchair exercise'	~~3 minutes~~
In bed: 'Relax to sleep'	2 minutes

Total 15 minutes

Fifteen minutes is the minimum time these exercises can be done in, but any of the routines may be repeated. If the 'Energising exercise' can be repeated in the afternoon or evening, so much the better. But if done only once a day with Coué's words — which need not be spoken aloud — the impulse has been sent out to the body to function better. I will now describe the exercises.

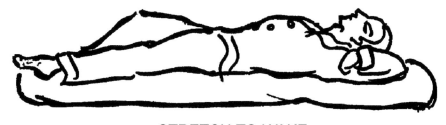

STRETCH TO WAKE

Remove pillow to lie flat on bed. Place the backs of both hands — relaxed — on each side of the neck, behind the ears, elbows above head.

Stretch the right elbow UP and the right leg DOWN, drawing left hip UP, and keeping the knee relaxed. Breathe IN as you stretch, then relax as you breathe OUT.

Repeat reversed stretching left side. Then do four quick stretches. Repeat routine until fully awake.

ENERGISING EXERCISES

These can be done on getting up and at any time during the day. The whole routine is done facing in the same direction but some figures are drawn in side view to make positions clearer.

ENERGISING EXERCISE 1

(a) Breathe and Contract
Can be done to music. Using Basic Breathing, breathe IN for Bars 1 and 2, breathe OUT for Bars 3 and 4.

BAR 1 'Breathe in the good': arms out sideways, palms forward.

BAR 2 'Assimilate': hold position, still breathing in.

BAR 3 'Breathe out the bad': place tips of fingers on sides of lower abdomen.

BAR 4 'Eliminate': arms out sideways, backs of hands forward. REPEAT EXACTLY.

(b) Stretch and Relax
Time and breathing as in previous 4 bars, but more movements in each bar.

BAR 1 'Stretch stretch': on 1st beat join palms of hands in front of, and close to the body; stretch above head to 2nd beat. On 3rd beat step sideways, taking whole of weight on to *right* foot, while bending body to the *left*. Reverse exactly, taking weight on to *left* foot, and bending body to the *right*.

BAR 2 'The spine extend': taking weight on both feet, keep hands together and stretch arms above head on 1st and 2nd beats. Part hands so that arms form a V shape. Arch back on 3rd beat; hold for 4th beat.

BAR 3 'Let go, relax': on 1st beat relax neck, wrists and elbows; on 2nd beat drop hands and relax upper spine.

BAR 4 'At waistline bend': continue relaxation to lumbar region only. Do not try to reach the ground as this involves flexion at the hip joint. REPEAT EXACTLY.

EACH OF THE ABOVE ROUTINES SHOULD BE REPEATED ONCE.

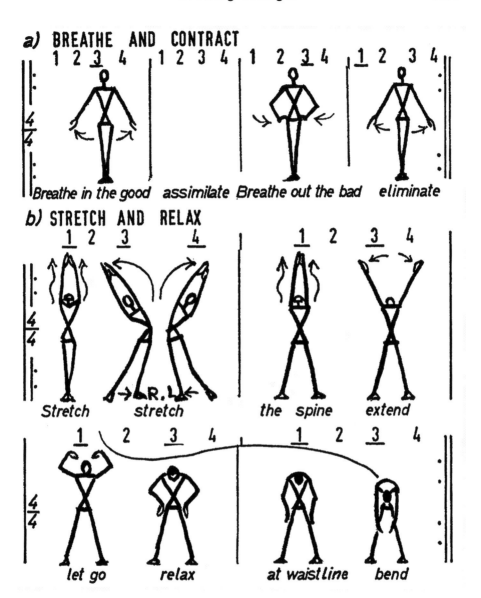

a) BREATHE AND CONTRACT

Breathe in the good   assimilate   Breathe out the bad   eliminate

b) STRETCH AND RELAX

Stretch   stretch   the spine   extend

let go   relax   at waistline   bend

ENERGISING EXERCISE 2

Thoracic movements to improve spinal mobility

Time: 4 beats in a bar. Breathing synchronised — 4 IN, 4 OUT throughout.

(a) Lateral — (double side flexion)

Starting position: wide stride, feet straight to fix pelvis. Elbows bent at shoulder level, hands palms down close to chest.

BAR 1 'Every day and in every way': 1st beat carry thorax to *right*, and a little further on 2nd beat. 3rd and 4th beats repeat above taking thorax to *left*.

BAR 2 'I am getting better and better': repeat BAR 1 but in double time, taking thorax right, left, right, left.

(b) Flexion and Extension

BAR 1 'Every day and in every way': 1st beat flex spine at lumbar region, head up, dorsal spine flat. Hold for 2nd beat. 3rd beat arch the back, stretching arms forward for balance, chin on chest. Hold for 4th beat.

BAR 2 'I function better and better': repeat BAR 1 in double time, bending at waist forward, back, forward, back.

(c) Rotation

BAR 1 'Every day and in every way': 1st beat twist thorax to *right*; 2nd beat twist a little further round, 3rd and 4th beats repeat above, twisting thorax to *left*.

BAR 2 'I do better and better': twisting thorax right, left, right, left.

(d) Side Flexion

BAR 1 'Every day and in every way': placing hands on top of head, 1st beat without moving feet, transfer all the weight on to the *right* foot, bending body to *left*, left leg relaxed. Hold for 2nd beat. 3rd beat, transfer all weight on to *left* foot, bending body to *right*.

BAR 2 'I think better and better': repeat BAR 1 in double time, transferring weight, right, left, right, left.

(a), (b), (c) and (d) SHOULD EACH BE DONE FOUR TIMES.

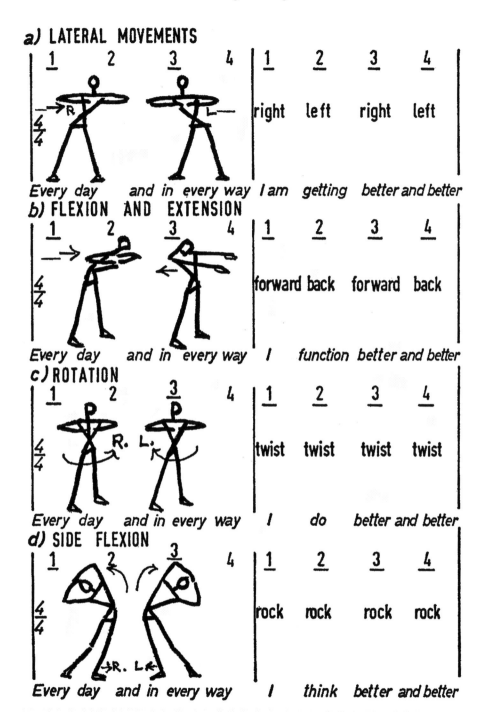

a) LATERAL MOVEMENTS

1	2	3	4
right	left	right	left

Every day   and in every way I am getting better and better

b) FLEXION AND EXTENSION

1	2	3	4
forward	back	forward	back

Every day   and in every way I   function better and better

c) ROTATION

1	2	3	4
twist	twist	twist	twist

Every day   and in every way   I   do   better and better

d) SIDE FLEXION

1	2	3	4
rock	rock	rock	rock

Every day   and in every way   I   think better and better

ENERGISING EXERCISE 3

(a) Breathe and Contract

Incorporates tilting of the pelvis. Time: 4 beats in a bar; Basic Breathing, IN for Bars 1 and 2, OUT for Bars 3 and 4.

BAR 1 'Breathe in the good': arms out sideways, pelvis back.

BAR 2 'Assimilate': hold position, still breathing in.

BAR 3 'Breathe out the bad': place tips of fingers on sides of lower abdomen, thumbs behind hip bone, tilting pelvis forward.

BAR 4 'Eliminate': hold this position, still breathing out.

REPEAT EXACTLY.

(b) Stretch and Relax

With full flexion of the spine and hip joints. Time and breathing: as in previous 4 bars, but more movements in each bar.

BAR 1 'Stretch, stretch': on 1st beat, joining palms in front of body, stretch straight up above head on 2nd beat. On 3rd beat, stretch right arm still further up; on 4th beat stretch up the left arm.

BAR 2 'The spine extend': 1st and 2nd beats, join palms above head; 3rd beat, part hands a little, still stretching up. Let head drop back.

BAR 3 'Reach out, relax': 1st beat, reach forward. 2nd beat, begin relaxation; 3rd and 4th beats, continue relaxation.

BAR 4 'And downward bend': relax whole spine, hip joints, and arms completely until fingers touch floor.

a) BREATHE AND CONTRACT

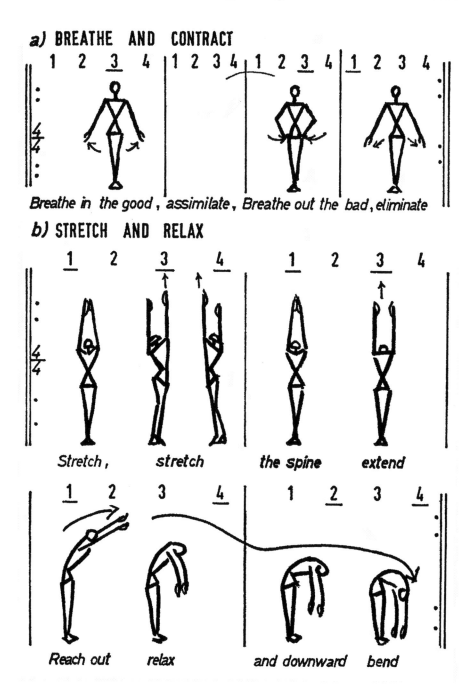

Breathe in the good, assimilate, Breathe out the bad, eliminate

b) STRETCH AND RELAX

Stretch,   stretch   the spine   extend

Reach out   relax   and downward   bend

ENERGISING EXERCISE 4

Pelvic Movements to Improve Spinal Mobility

Time and Breathing: as in Energising Exercise 2. Feet together throughout, knees slightly relaxed, to allow full range of pelvic movement. Starting position: arms sideways, elbows flexed on frontal plane, hands about a yard apart, away from hips, palms down, fists loosely clenched.

(a) Lateral — (double side flexion).

BAR 1 'Every day and in every way': 1st beat, carry pelvis to *right*, 2nd beat, move pelvis a little further. 3rd and 4th beats, repeat above, taking pelvis to the *left*.

BAR 2 'I am getting better and better': repeat BAR 1 but in double time, right, left, right left.

(b) Flexion and Extension

Place hands low on hips, fingers in front, thumbs behind.

BAR 1 'Every day and in every way': 1st beat, flex lumbar spine, tilting pelvis forward; hold for 2nd beat. 3rd beat, extend lumbar spine, tilting pelvis backwards; hold for 4th beat.

BAR 2 'I function better and better': repeat BAR 1 in double time, tilting forward, back, forward, back.

(c) Rotation

Hands in front, loosely clenched, almost touching, elbows forward. Try not to move hands or shoulders while twisting pelvis.

BAR 1 'Every day and in every way': 1st beat, twist pelvis to *right*; 2nd beat, twist a little further round. 3rd and 4th beats, repeat above twisting pelvis to *left*.

BAR 2 'I do better and better': repeat BAR 1 in double time, right, left, right left.

(d) Side Flexion

Arms crossed relaxed over top of head.

BAR 1 'Every day and in every way': 1st beat, pull up right hip, hold for 2nd beat. 3rd and 4th beats, pull up left hip.

BAR 2 'I think better and better': repeat BAR 1 in double time, pulling up right, left, right, left.

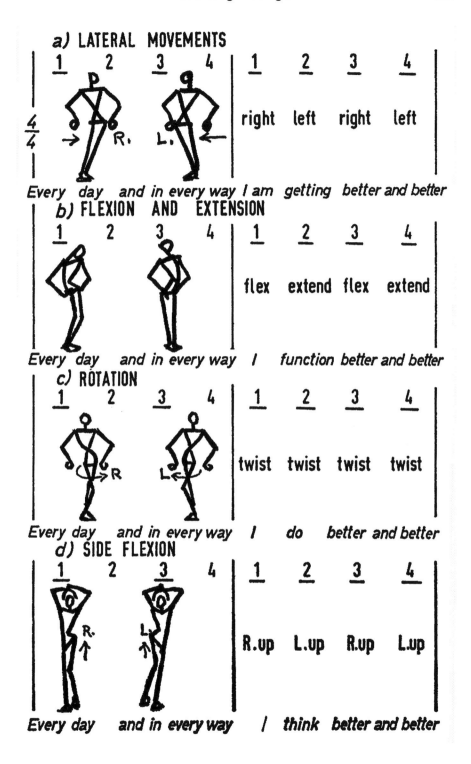

a) LATERAL MOVEMENTS

1	2	3	4	1	2	3	4
				right	left	right	left

Every day and in every way I am getting better and better

b) FLEXION AND EXTENSION

1	2	3	4	1	2	3	4
				flex	extend	flex	extend

Every day and in every way I function better and better

c) ROTATION

1	2	3	4	1	2	3	4
				twist	twist	twist	twist

Every day and in every way I do better and better

d) SIDE FLEXION

1	2	3	4	1	2	3	4
				R.up	L.up	R.up	L.up

Every day and in every way I think better and better

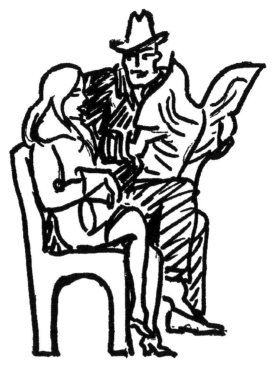

INVISIBLE EXERCISE

This can be done sitting — wherever you happen to be — with both feet firmly planted on the floor. Arms, hands and head may be in any position but should be kept still throughout.

(a) Basic Breathing.

This can be done anywhere, at any time, without being at all noticeable, if on breathing out the lips are only slightly parted, letting the air escape soundlessly. Or the air may be breathed out through the nose. The abdomen should, as always, be firmly drawn in, as this movement is invisible.

(b) Alternate Foot Lifting

First take a deep breath through the nose. While breathing out, lift the right foot just off the ground (one inch) keeping the knee bent. Repeat this time by raising the left foot. Lifting the foot, however small the movement, uses the recti muscles of the abdomen, together with the transverses. Repeat as often as time will allow.

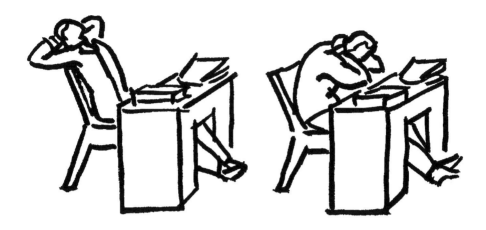

RENEWING EXERCISE

When energy begins to flag, a few deep breaths help enormously.

(a) Basic Breathing

Sit well back in your chair or lean forward, elbows on your desk. The pulling in of the abdomen on expiration is the most important part, as this helps the return of the blood to the heart, and also aids digestion.

(b) Stretch and Relax

Clasp the hands behind the neck, take a deep breath while arching the back against your chair, pressing the elbows backwards. While breathing out, relax the whole spine, letting the elbows come forward as you draw in the abdomen.

(c) Thoracic Mobility: Rotation

Rest hands on upper chest wall, elbows sideways at shoulder level. Breathe in deeply, facing forward. While breathing out, turn thorax to the right as far as possible. The head must be kept facing forward so that the chin is pointing over the left shoulder, the abdomen drawn in. Repeat exactly, but turning to the left.

(d) Lateral Movement

Rest your hands on the arms of the chair: or, if none, on the sides of the seat. Breathe in deeply, stretching body upward. When breathing out, carry the thorax to the right as far as possible, drawing in the abdomen. Repeat exactly, but taking thorax to the left. All movements should be repeated four or eight times.

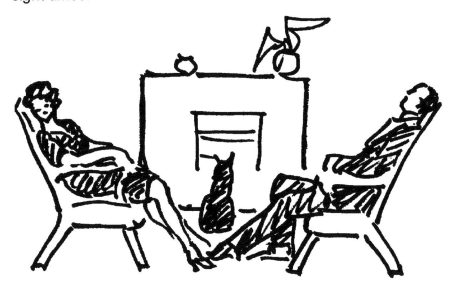

ARMCHAIR EXERCISE

A solid, well-padded armchair is the most comfortable, but a modern-style chair with arms can be used if it is strong enough and steady. In order to derive any benefit, it is essential to be really comfortable and relaxed. Pad the chair with cushions if necessary, the first objectives being relaxation and enjoyment. Do the exercise in your own time, but as slowly as you can with comfort. Breathe in deeply, but don't worry too much about abdominal contraction — if you do it easily that is fine, but the whole routine should be pleasant to do, and make you feel rested.

(a) Stretch, Stretch

Hold the top of the back of the chair, elbows above your head. Do the stretching you did in the first exercise, but at the

STRETCH — STRETCH

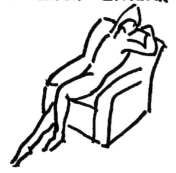

ROTATION

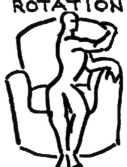

SIDE FLEXION

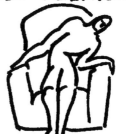

BREATHE & RELAX

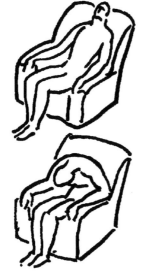

TWIST & STRETCH

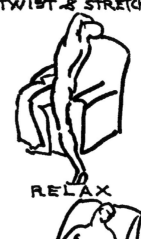

MOBILITY—LATERAL

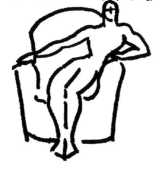

RELAX

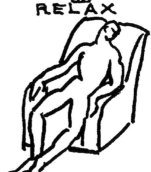

same time pull on the back of the chair to get an extra stretch, which is refreshing and helps to relax.

(b) Breathe and Relax

Breathe in deeply, Extend the spine by arching the back against the chair, arms out sideways. Breathe out, flexing spine and letting arms fall forward, completely relaxed.

(c) Lateral Movement

Place hands on arms of chair, breathe in deeply, stretching body upwards. While breathing out, take the right elbow to the side, fully flexed, and carry the thorax to the right, extending the left arm. Repeat, but this time carry the thorax to the left.

(d) Rotation

Breathe in deeply, hands resting on arms of chair. While breathing out, turn thorax to the right — without moving legs and feet — and take the left arm across and hold side of chair back, pulling gently to assist the rotation of the trunk. Repeat exactly to the left.

(e) Side Flexion

Breathe in deeply, hands resting on arms of chair. While breathing out, bend sideways to the right, flexing right elbow. Legs and feet should not move. Repeat bending to the left.

(f) Twist, Stretch and Relax

In this case the stretching movement is done while breathing in. Turning to the right, hold top corner of chair back with left hand, elbow flexed, while stretching back the left leg. This stretches the intercostals muscles on that side, facilitating the expansion of that lung. While breathing out, roll on to the back, relaxing the whole body completely, letting the arms and legs fall into easy positions. Repeat exactly to the left.

RELAX TO SLEEP

This routine is the one exception to breathing out through the mouth and pulling in the abdomen, because there should be no conscious effort. Breathe in and out through the nose, at your normal pace.

(a) Stretch

Begin with the morning's 'Stretch to wake' exercise, but take it easily. The slight stretch relieves tension, helps the circulation and makes relaxation easier.

(b) Gently Stretch, Fully Relax

Lie comfortably on your back, feet slightly apart, knees relaxed, arms resting loosely at your sides.

Breathe in slowly and easily, gently stretching from the top of your head to the tips of your toes and fingers, just feel conscious of your muscles.

As you breathe out, let go and relax completely, feel your whole body heavy, imagine it is falling right through the mattress.

Do this four to eight times, but gradually stretching less and relaxing more, until all effort ceases. Then roll over into your most comfortable position and sink into a deep and restful sleep

SPECIAL EXERCISES

1 : IRONING OUT THE SPINE

This is the best routine for correcting round back, poking head and middle-age stoop. To get results it must be done on a hard flat surface — preferably a wood or tiled floor. If carpeted, the floor should be comfortable enough, but on a tiled or concrete floor a slightly padded beach mattress may be used.

The routine consists of doing Basic Breathing in 'crook lying' — with the arms in eight different positions, as shown in the diagrams over the page. On breathing out, the abdominal contraction should be emphasised, pressing the lumbar spine firmly on to the floor. Changing the position of the arms brings the pressure on different parts of the spine from the waist up.

Take four deep breaths in each position without moving the arms, trying to keep them and the backs of the hands in contact with the floor throughout. Having got to the eighth position, the hardest — the arms stretched straight above the head, but still on the floor — repeat exactly, but this time work downwards, as indicated by the numbers on the diagrams over the page.

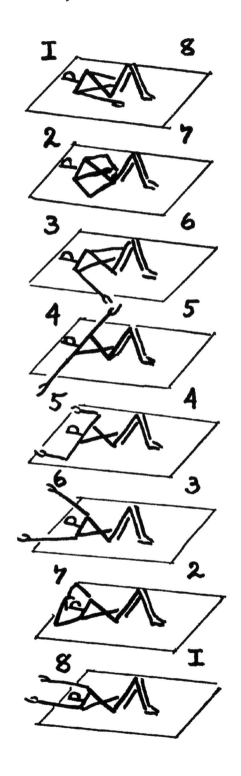

2 : HIP ROLLING

This is the most obvious exercise for reducing, as the pressure of the floor on thighs and hips helps break down the fatty tissues. Clearly, this exercise must be done on a hard flat surface. Basic Breathing should be practised constantly since the oxygen in the blood helps burn up the excess fat in the tissues. Take the crook-lying position, but with the arms extended at shoulder level, backs of the hands on the floor.

(a) Drop knees to floor on *right* for a count of two; repeat, but dropping knees to the floor on *left*.

(b) As above but at twice the speed, taking knees over to right, left, right, left. Arms and shoulders should not move, and should be in contact with the floor throughout.

(c) Draw up knees until the heels touch the thighs. Then repeat a) but this time keep the knees at hip level.

(d) Draw up the knees until they almost touch your chest. Then repeat (a), keeping knees at chest level.

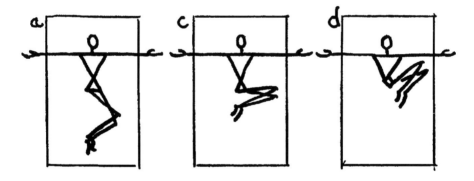

3 : NECK MOBILITY

These exercises can be done to music, as they are most effective when done rhythmically.

(a) Flexion and Extension

BAR 1 Drop head forward for 1st beat, hold for 2nd. Drop head backwards on 3rd beat, hold for 4th.

BAR 2 Repeat above at twice the speed, dropping head forward, back, forward, back.

(b) Rotation

BAR 1 Turn head to the right for 1st beat, hold for 2nd. Turn head to the left for 3rd beat, hold for 4th.

BAR 2 Repeat above at twice the speed, turning head right, left, right, left.

(c) Side Flexion

BAR 1 Drop head on to right shoulder on 1st beat, hold for 2nd. Drop head on to left shoulder for 3rd beat, hold for 4th.

BAR 2 Repeat above at twice the speed, to right, left, right, left.

(d) Circling

This combines all the movements and is an excellent exercise. However, it should be tried very gently at first for it can cause giddiness if the liver is congested, or if there is something wrong with the eyes.

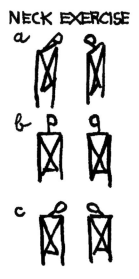

NECK EXERCISE

4 : EYE MOBILITY

This exercise includes all the movements of which the eye is capable, some of which are only rarely used. After middle age, most people only look up, down or straight ahead. If asked to look at something at the side, they turn their heads in that direction. They rarely look to the corners, or circle the eyes completely. Yet all the movements of which the eyes are capable are necessary to keep the eye muscles in tone, and to maintain the required blood supply.

To do these exercises, it is important to be relaxed and comfortable. You may sit, recline or lie, but make sure the head is well supported and the neck relaxed. Only the eyes must move. Watch that the body and limbs are not tensed. The movements are arranged to fit a time of three beats in a bar (see next page).

(a) Blink the eyes for six beats, close for six beats. Do this four times.

(b) Look to corners as shown in the diagram numbers 1-9, starting at top *right*-hand corner. Close eyes for a count of three (numbers 10,11 and 12). Then repeat, starting at top *left* hand corner.

(c) Blink eyes for six beats, squeeze shut for six beats. Repeat this four times.

(d) Look up and down: follow diagram numbers 1-9. Squeeze shut for numbers 10,11 and 12

(e) Blink eyes for six beats, squeeze shut for six beats. Repeat this four times.

(f) Look from side to side: Follow diagram numbers 1-9. Squeeze shut for numbers 10,11 and 12.

(g) Long blink: keeping eyes fixed on one spot, blink without stopping for 48 beats.

(h) First look up, then circle eyes to the right twice (numbers 1-9). Close for 10,11 and 12. Repeat, circling eyes to the left. Close eyes to relax them at finish.

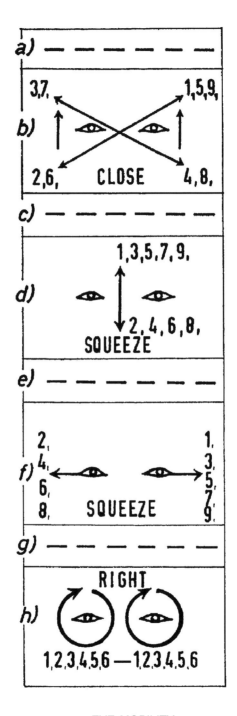

EYE MOBILITY

5 : SECRET EXERCISE

So called because no one should ever see you do it. Do not even look at yourself, it is too depressing. It is important to keep the muscles of the face and of the neck in tone, and to improve the blood supply to the skin. It helps if gentle sounds are made as indicated.

    (a) 00 — ee
    (b) oo — or
    (c) oo — for
    (d) oo — wah

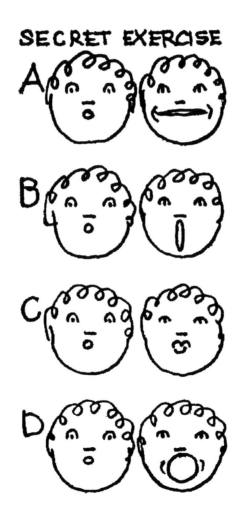

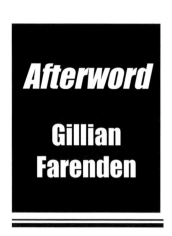

Afterword

Gillian Farenden

THE FIRST EDITION OF MY LIFE IN MOVEMENT, which you have been reading up to now, was published in 1969. In the years following, Margaret Morris Movement was to continue as it had since 1961 (the year of J.D. Fergusson's death and the closure of the London and Glasgow schools) as an informal organisation of teachers and dancers, working and performing, scattered through the UK and abroad. Its annual Summer Schools brought these members together once a year, and contacts were held together primarily by the efforts of Isabel Jeayes, who had kept the membership records and whose newsletters kept both teachers and members in touch.

Margaret Morris herself concentrated increasingly on promoting the art work of her husband, J. D. Fergusson, and on her own writing. In 1972, *Creation in Dance and Life* was published by Peter Owen, publishers of her first book, further establishing her method of movement teaching and improvisation, and two years later *The Art of J. D. Fergusson — A Biased Biography* appeared. The interesting subtitle of this book revealed Margaret's own admission that her view of her husband's work could hardly be called objective; nevertheless, the work gave a close and personal insight into his life and work and an appraisal of his artistic achievement.

During these years she also worked on the manuscript for a book on improvisation, which Peter Owen wanted to publish as a sequel to *Creation in Dance and Life* to complete the scope of her movement teaching. This work had been started much earlier — however, it was presumed lost in the war as neither Margaret nor Isabel, keeper of all records and archives, could locate it. So, undaunted, she began to re-write this book, which unfortunately remained unpublished.

In 1973 'the lady from the BBC' was able to make her own television film, a project made possible by a grant from the Scottish Arts Council and Educational Films of Scotland. However, she was unhappy about the finished product, a demonstration and explanation of the exercises showing the full range of her training method. The money available had only been sufficient for the hire of one small studio in Glasgow and one static camera, which sadly limited the performance of dance and, more important, caused one aspect of her work — the improvisation sessions showing Jim Hastie performing with Margaret herself — to be omitted entirely. Although shown on television, the film was not considered by Margaret to be a worthy record of her work. However, as always, she was not deterred by this set-back but simply put it aside and carried on.

Meanwhile she had set up the J. D. Fergusson Art Foundation and organised exhibitions of his work, offering the collection to galleries, and achieving ultimately a permanent collection at the Round House, provided by Perth and Kinross District Council. (This was later to be converted into the Fergusson Gallery, with its own keeper, opened in March 1992.) A BBC film of J. D. Fergusson's work was made in 1976, narrated by Margaret herself. Thus her efforts during these years achieved for her husband an increase of recognition and appreciation, and established the name of a significant Scottish artist.

However she did not neglect her own life's work. Margaret continued to oversee the continuing dance and teacher training by visiting the annual Summer Schools, at which in 1973 Jim Hastie taught after an absence (at Culham College in

Oxfordshire). At that time Margaret's former dancer was working with the Scottish Ballet and Scottish Opera in Glasgow, and this Summer School marked the beginning of a closer involvement for Jim which was to be of significance for the continuation of Margaret Morris Movement. He became even more involved in 1975, when Isabel handed over to him the list of approximately 100 teachers and members which she had been keeping since the closure of the schools, as well as £200 in cash representing the total funds of M.M.M.. Jim took a small office in Hanover Street in Edinburgh, from where he issued a newsletter to members printed on a second hand duplicator — and thus took over the organisation of the Movement, not knowing then that this was to become his full-time occupation for the next decades and ultimately his life's work.

The same year he made a visit to Switzerland, where M.M.M. was being taught by Suzanne Chapuis and Constance Ochsenbein; this was to be the first of many regular trips abroad which were to shape the future of M.M.M.. Jim's work was assisted by the first grant of funds from the Sports Council in 1976, a development grant, to be followed by an administration grant in 1977.

That year Margaret made her last visit to a Summer School (by now held at Balls Park in Hertford), as the following year her health forced her to give up her London and Glasgow flats and move to Sussex, where she lived with two cousins, first with Katherine and then with Joan. After Joan's death she moved temporarily into a home, but returned to Glasgow in 1979, where a year later she 'died with her boots on' — still active to the last. She had seen her Movement grow in the last decade of her life — M.M.M. was already in existence in Switzerland, France, Canada, South Africa, Germany and Japan (Jim Hastie's first visit there taking place shortly after her death). She had ensured the continuation of M.M.M. in and outside the UK, had committed her theories and philosophy and the principles of her movement teaching to paper; and had achieved recognition of her husband's work. She could leave this world knowing that she had given — and would continue to give through Margaret

Morris Movement in the future.

The late seventies and early eighties were years of consolidation and expansion for the International Association of Margaret Morris Movement. Jim Hastie's first visit to France (1976), Canada (1977) where Iris Holdup had started classes in 1951, Germany (1978) and Japan (1980), together with regular trips to Switzerland, engendered a tremendous increase of enthusiasm for the Movement in these countries, which spilled over into the UK and manifested itself most obviously at the annual Summer Schools with their growing numbers of attendees each year. Jim had by now taken over as Administrator and Director of Training, assisted by a full-time administration grant from the Sports Council which was awarded for the first time in 1980.

A most significant contributory factor to the expansion of M.M.M. during these years was the establishment of the M.M.M. Centre at Biggin Hill, Kent, officially opened in May 1982 by Olive Newson, Senior Executive Officer of the Sports Council. The house and gardens at Sunningvale Avenue, Biggin Hill, had been bequeathed to M.M.M. by Nina Hosali, and money had been accumulated over a period of years by fund-raising activities and donations including a special grant from the Sports Council. At the opening ceremony a celebratory performance of exercises and dances was given in the newly erected studio (also containing a classroom, shower facilities and kitchen, and able to accommodate up to twenty dancers for courses and seminars). Nina Hosali's house became living quarters and community centre for the quickly established week-long intensive courses and weekend seminars. Thus, twenty-one years after the closure of the last full-time schools, M.M.M. once more had a permanent centre of activitiy and of learning.

Although the M.M.M. Centre was not a full-time training school, it did (together with the annual Summer Schools) provide an essential opportunity for dance training and teaching courses which further assisted growth during these years. Add to this the publication of the 'Colour Manuals' describing the exercises contained in each grade of the system, which were essential tools for teachers in training, and the thorough, well-founded base for the continuation of M.M.M. becomes visible — an aspect which distinguished M.M.M. then, as it does today, from many other forms of movement and activity, which did not and will not stand the test of time. The first of the Colour Manuals for the Basic exercises had been written by Jim Hastie and illustrated by Robin Anderson back in 1961/62 immediately after the schools closed, and was first published in 1963; however, for later editions the illustrations were omitted, as it was feared this would lead to the practice of M.M.M. by people without proper training and qualifications, who simply 'worked from the book' — thus possibly discrediting the system by wrong interpretation and bad or unqualified teaching. Jim continued the series of books for the colours from White to Dark Pink, making seven in all, including Basic, in the years up to 1986, thus greatly assisting the many teachers and performers who trained during these years and since.

In 1977 the M.M.M. Movement Therapy Course was re-instated, successful completion of which qualified M.M.M. teachers to use Margaret's system to work with the elderly, the physically and mentally impaired and those in rehabilitation after illness or accident. Additional books were prepared for the M.M.M. Children's Grades and Health Play, thus completing the range of teaching manuals for M.M.M. qualifications.

The Sports Council's grant was the essential foundation for this work and growth period, as it enabled Jim Hastie to devote his time and energy fully to the development and propagation of M.M.M.. From his office in Edinburgh he issued the twice-yearly magazine and kept the records of members and teachers, whose numbers were by now growing rapidly in all countries. Soon fully-recognised national organisations were established, affiliated to the International Association, with contractual agreements regulating their status and activity in relation to the parent organisation. In most cases M.M.M. had been present in these countries as early as before the war, but with the establishment of the national organisations M.M.M. gained a new public status and acknowledgement in the world of dance

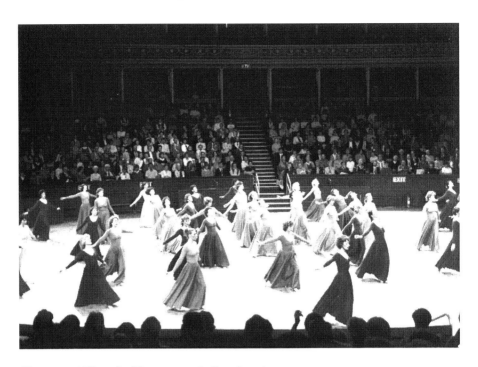

**Margaret Morris Movement display team,
Royal Albert Hall, 1985.**

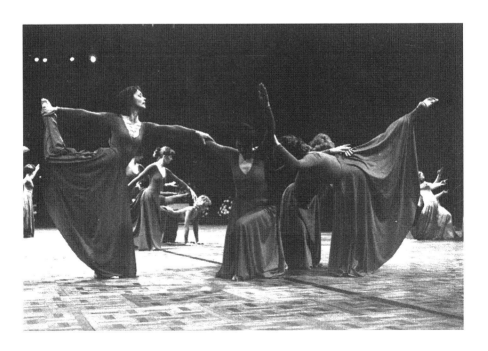

and recreational movement. A worldwide international network emerged.

In the UK too an increase in public exposure took place in the eighties, with participation at national events, at conferences, and at M.M.M.'s own festivals celebrating milestones in the history of the movement. Among these celebratory events was the performance commemorating the 70th Anniversary of the M.M.M. technique, held at Balls Park, Hertford, during the Summer School of 1980. This consisted of revivals of Margaret's own choreography danced in the original costumes, which had been safely stored. Five years later a similar performance for the 75th Anniversary showed an expanded programme of dances and a 'tableau vivant' using the original costumes from further dances, and the same year the first M.M.M. Festival was held at the Wembley Conference Centre in London. The reconstructed dances were also peformed twice in Scotland, by M.M.M. dancers and members of the Scottish Ballet, with whom Jim Hastie retained close links even after giving up his work there in favour of M.M.M.. Thus M.M.M. helped to raise funds for the completion of the Robin Anderson Theatre in Glasgow by the joint performance in 1986. The second performance two years later in the year of the Garden Festival in Glasgow was held at the King's Theatre, with musicians and singers, and using full orchestral scores from the original performances which had been recovered shortly before. At this event the dance 'Gloxinia', dating from 1924, was performed by Barbara West, who had reconstructed the choreography entirely from the original M.M.M. notation.

Through its close connection with the Sports Council M.M.M. was invited to participate at national events organised by the Central Council for Physical Recreation (CCPR) and by the Keep Fit Association. These events gave M.M.M. dancers the chance to appear at the Royal Albert Hall in London — with dances and demonstrations peformed by teachers and pupils from across the UK (in 1980 at the KFA Festival, 1985 at the Golden Jubilee of the CCPR, and 1987 for Age Concern).

Recognition of Margaret Morris and her work was also

demonstrated by participation at the conference held at the University of Surrey in 1983 entitled 'Early Pioneers of Modern Dance', which was concerned with the work of Ruby Ginner, Madge Atkinson and — Margaret Morris. And in 1989 a comparison of notation systems was published by Ann Hutchinson Guest, dealing amongst others with the system devised by Margaret Morris. Several publications of this decade contributed to the record of Margaret's work in dance and art, among them the Third Eye Centre's book *MM Drawings and Designs and the Glasgow Years* and the catalogue of the art exhibition 'Colour, Rhythm and Dance' with works by J. D. Fergusson and members of his circle. This exhibition was shown in Scotland and France in 1985, following a successful showing at the Cyril Gerber Fine Art Gallery a year earlier of Margaret Morris's own art work.

Meanwhile the number of foreign countries where M.M.M. was being taught was constantly growing — in 1984 M.M.M. was introduced on the Ivory Coast (brought there by Sonja Couzy, who had been reponsible for its introduction to Germany and Japan), classes in Sweden and Malta were also established, and in Australia in 1988, when Jill Perry went to live in Perth. The international network was spreading out, and M.M.M. was true to its name — the International Association of M.M.M..

1991 was a year of celebration. Three major events were organised to commemorate the centenary of Margaret Morris's birth. A new exhibition of Margaret's drawings, paintings and designs was shown at the Cyril Gerber Fine Art Gallery in Glasgow, and a Festival of Dance held again at Wembley Conference Centre, sponsored by the Hosali Foundation, at which not only British but also foreign groups took part. At the Summer School of that year an extended programme of historical dances in costume, including the reconstructed 'Gloxinia' and the 'tableau vivant' to display further original costumes was put on — at which the guest of honour was Olive Newson, meanwhile retired from her position with the Sports Council, but remaining a friend of M.M.M..

The Festival performance at Wembley initiated a series of annual events entitled 'Dance for All', which began in 1992 with a performance in Exeter and continues each year at different regional theatres throughout England. This showcase, performed by groups from all UK regions, until 2000 under the overall organisation of Kathleen Watkinson, aimed to demonstrate to an outside audience as well as to M.M.M. members and friends the wide range of activity taking place under the M.M.M. umbrella — children's dances, items by teenagers and young adults, the more mature, and senior citizens. Performers were not professionals but 'ordinary' class members, and groups of performers and audience travelled from all over the country to the venue for a full day of rehearsals and performance.

M.M.M.'s participation at CCPR events and festivals continued, with the KFA Festival in 1992 at the National Exhibition Centre Arena in Birmingham, and once more to the Royal Albert Hall for the CCPR's diamond jubilee in 1995. Although there was no permanent dance group to perform at these events, the number of trained teachers and active dancers in the UK had grown so as to enable a team to be brought together which, because of the uniform training and standard of performance, was able to put together a cohesive, harmonious performance in a short space of rehearsal time, under the direction of Jim Hastie. From this supply teams could be put together for demonstrations and workshop classes at other national events of the nineties, for example Dance UK, Blitz, exhibitions at Earls Court or the Olympia arena, or at the Barbican conference centre in London. The reason for the harmony in performance was the constant common factor of training achieved by the M.M.M. system with its carefully built-up syllabus of exercises, and the network of meticulously trained teachers who up to the present day are still examined by those trained by Margaret herself, or by her immediate successor, Director of Training Jim Hastie. Thus a harmony is demonstrated which, in spite of this common background, still leaves ample scope for the individual to interpret, to express and to show his/her individual creative self in performance.

Today, after the end of the century during most of which Margaret Morris lived and worked, M.M.M. is still expanding in its range of activity and gaining the acceptance and recognition it truly deserves, especially in the field of education. Margaret wrote in *Margaret Morris Dancing* (1925) :

> 'The only reasonable means of helping young children to develop is through the artistic or creative side. ... Every human being, unless he is devoid of creative possibilities, is to some extent potentially an artist. The time when the creative instinct usually takes artistic form most strongly is in childhood.... By educating children first through the study and observation of movement, colour and sound, they are given a natural outlet for ideas and emotions; and by discovering a means of expression, the repressions that are the cause of so many disorders in later life can for the most part be avoided.'

Today in the educational system of most European countries, this emphasis is being re-addressed after a period of concentration on academic achievement to the detriment of the individual creative development of the child. M.M.M. is active in this development; through its programme "Dance Action for Youth" M.M.M. offers teachers in schools a training syllabus to help them guide pupils into this important aspect of their education. Thus after nearly a century of Margaret Morris Movement, the system has now arrived, in a number of countries, where Margaret intended it to be: integrated into the school educational programme of all young people.

This is not only the future of M.M.M., but where it is already fulfilling a valuable role today. Where it will go from here is the story for the next edition of this book to tell. But M.M.M. will most certainly continue, as it has so much to offer and is so relevant for all sections of our society, today and in years to come.

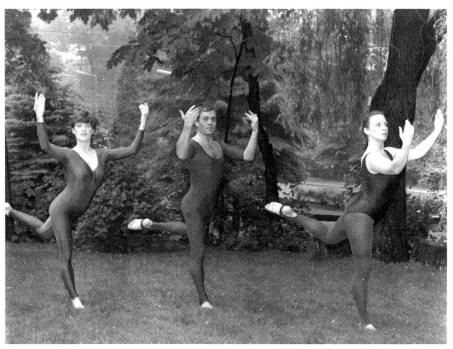

(Above) Beverley Currie, Jim Hastie and Janet Houselander at the Canadian Summer School; (below) Class at the 2002 Summer School, Wall Hall, Hertfordshire.
Photograph: Julian Rose.

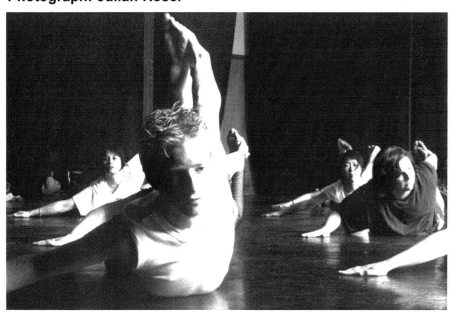

Bibliographical References

1.Margaret Morris, *My Galsworthy Story* (Peter Owen, 1967).

2. Margaret Morris, *The Notation of Movement*
(Routledge & Kegan Paul, 1928).

2a. Margaret Morris and Hans Falkner, *Skiing Exercises*
(Heinemann, 1934).

3. Margaret Morris in collaboration with M. Randell,
Maternity and Post Operative Exercises (Heinemann 1936).

4. Margaret Morris in collaboration with Suzanne Lenglen,
Tennis by Simple Exercises (Heinemann, 1937).

5. Margaret Morris, *Basic Physical Training* (Heinemann, 1937).

6. Margaret Morris with photographs by Fred Daniels,
Margaret Morris Dancing (Routledge & Kegan Paul, 1925).

7. Ann Hutchinson, *Labanotation* (Phoenix House, 1954).

8. F. A. Hornibrook, *The Culture of the Abdomen*
(Heinemann, 1924).

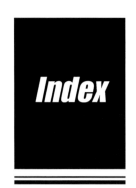

Index

Adlard, Betsy, 65
Adler, Jankel, 106
Ailey, Alvin, 160
Ainsworth, Elizabeth, 48
Allen, Maud, 32
Anderson, Robin, 125, 151, 225, 227
Archer, David, 106, 107
Atkinson, Madge, 228
Arnott, James, 90
Austin, 'Bunny', 86

Baddeley, Angela, 23, 28, 121
Baddeley, Hermione, 28
Baddeley, Muriel, 28
Bain, Donald, 103, 126
Baird, Sir Dugald, 92, 93
Baker, Noel, 131
Bannister, Winifred, 108, 124
Bantock, Granville, 34
Banzie, Marie de, 103
Barham, Gwen, 79, 80
Barker-Mill, Elsa, 29
Bax, Arnold, 34
Baxter, Stanley, 103
Baylis, Lilian, 157

Beard, Paul, 121
Benesh, 153, 154
Benson, Frank & Mrs, 8
Beaumont, Comte de, 40
Bilsland, Lord and Lady, 123
Bligh, Jasmine, 94
Blum, Odette, 103
Borotra, Jean, 71
Boughton, Rutland, 22, 23, 33
Bradford, Hugh, 93
Brema, Marie, 11
Bridie, James, 104
Bristow, Mr, 55
Bruce, Veronica, 126
Buckmaster, Lady, 134
Burleigh, Lord, 133
Burns, Robert, 129
Burrowes, Leslie, 159
Bryant, Thelma, 103

Calvert, Phyllis, 48, 121, 122
Campbell, Mary, 115
Carpenter, Freddie, 110
Cassidy Claire, 98
Chapuis, Suzanne, 223
Chisholm, Erik, 100, 102, 108

Cholmondeley, Lady, 73, 91
Cholmondeley, Lord, 73, 83, 87, 91
Christian, John, 115
Clark, Kitty, 95
Cohen, Harriet, 34
Colquhoun, Robert, 163
Cooper, Gladys, 13
Cornock-Taylor, Anne, 98,131
Coton, A. V., 151
Couzy, Sonja, 228
Craig, Gordon, 156
Crosbie, William, 102
Crosfield, Lady, 86
Cruickshank, Stuart, 118, 120, 121

D'Albert, Eugene, 103
Daniels, Fred, 47
Dare, Marie, 126
D'Auban, John, 6, 8
Davidson, William, 27
Davison, Doreen, 36
Davison, George, 33, 36,
Dawkins, Kenneth, 126, 129
Diaghilev, Sergei, 21, 22, 103, 157
Dillon, Kathleen, 17, 23
Dolan, Sir Patrick, 99, 101
Doone, Rupert, 30
Duncan, Elizabeth, 64
Duncan, Isadora, 9, 159
Duncan, Raymond, 9, 10, 22, 147
Dunham, Katherine, 160

Eadie, Dennis, 13

Einert, Margaret, 92
Elder, Eleanor, 23, 121
Eliet, Dr, 95
Elmslie, Mr, 55
Epstein, Jacob, 25
Evans, Howard, 73, 74, 75

Fairbairn, Dr, 68
Falkner, Hans, 67, 95
Fergusson, Finlay & Meg, 120
Fergusson, J.D., 19-22, 24, 27, 34, 36, 37, 43, 79, 98-100, 104, 118, 121, 126, 221, 222, 228
Fergusson, Marjorie, 120
Findlay, Stuart, 102
Fitzgerald, Scott, 40
Fokine, Michael, 29, 157
Fraser, Kennedy, 81
Fraser, Mrs Kennedy, 81, 129
French, Lady, 123
Friedlander, Dr, 106
Frizell, J. B., 80
Frood, Millie, 125

Galsworthy, Ada, 11, 147
Galsworth, John, 11, 13, 17, 19, 147
Gates, Dorothy & Eric, 83
Gaye, Freda, 47
Gaye, Phoebe, 17, 47
Gem, A. H., 133
Gerber, Cyril, 228
Gielgud, John, 17
Gilmore, Avril, 44, 95
Ginner, Ruby, 11, 228
Girvan, George, 107

Godfrey, Dan, 23, 31
Goossens, Eugene, 25, 33, 34
Goossens, Leon, 159
Gopal, Ram, 115, 116, 133, 134
Gordon, Harry, 111
Graham, Martha, 64, 159, 161
Grant, Alexander, 62
Grant, Martha, 92
Greet, Ben, 6, 8
Grey, Beryl, 164
Gunn, James, 65
Gunson, Jocelyn, 65

Haines, Lett, 25
Halliday, Dr, 106
Harper, Roland, 86
Harrison, Ian, 162
Hastie, Jim, 125, 222-225, 227, 229
Henderson, Wight, 102
Herman, Josef, 102, 106
Hewlitt, Maurice, 17
Holbrook, Jackson, 19
Holdup, Iris, 224
Honeyman, T. J., 106
Hosali, Nina, 121, 224
Hutchinson-Guest, Ann, 151, 153, 154, 228
Hutton, Lois, 43

Iden, Rosalind, 28
Inverclyde, Lord, 123
Ireland, Kenneth, 118, 120

Jeayes, Isabel, 91, 92, 103, 121, 131, 221, 222
John, Augustus, 25

Jones, Sir Robert, 55
Jooss, Kurt, 159, 160
Joyce, James, 65

Karsavina, Tamara, 157
Kidd, Michael, 161
Kimmins, Mrs, 57, 58, 69

Laban, Rudolf von, 60, 147, 157
Lambert, Constant, 25
Lanchester, Elsa, 28
Lauder, Harry, 129
Laughton, Charles, 28
Lawson, Joan, 28
Lenglen, Suzanne, 71, 86
Levick, Dr Murray, 55, 56
Lewis, Wyndham, 25
Logan, Jimmy, 111
Lovelock, Dr Jack, 84

MacAulay, Angus, 162
MacBeth, Sylvia, 114, 118, 125
MacBryde, Robert, 162
McClure, Bruce, 107, 110, 111, 117, 126
McCombe, Mrs Norman, 123
Macdonald, Tom, 100
MacKellar, Kenneth, 110
Mackintosh, Charles Rennie, 26
Macintosh, Dr Stewart, 80, 81, 104, 105
Maclellan, William, 100
MacLeod, Kitty, 128
McNiell, Marian, 125
Macrae, Duncan, 111
Mansfield, Katharine, 25, 77, 78, 121

March, Dennis, 98
Massine, Leonid, 158, 162-164,
Matisse, Henri, 21
Maundrell, Miss F., 47
Maxwell, Sir John Stirling, 101
Middleton, Marjorie, 162
Millay, Edna St Vincent, 36
Mille, Agnes de, 161
Moonie, W.B., 123
Morris, Cedric, 25, 26
Morris, Joan, 223
Morris, Katherine, 223
Morrison, Angus, 28
Morrison, Kenneth, 126
Morton, John, 104
Murry, John Middleton, 25

Neill, Sheila, 126
Newson, Olive, 224, 228
Nijinsky, 147, 157, 158
Norton, Lady ('Peter'), 67, 75,

Ochsenbein, Constance, 223
Ogden, C. K., 60
Osterberg, Madame, 77
Ostrehan, Blanche, 28

Pagan, Isobel, 10
Paul, Kegan, 60, 146
Pavlova, Anna, 157
Peploe, S. J., 21, 98
Perry, Jill, 228
Picasso, Pablo, 19, 40
Pink, Dr Cyril, 29, 92
Pound, Ezra, 25
Pride, James, 156
Prost, Daniel & Rita, 96, 132

Rambert, Marie, 159, 162
Randell, Sister, 55, 62, 63,
    68, 81
Richardson, Philip, 120
Robbins, Jerome, 161
Rolla, Andrew, 103, 117
Rollier, Dr, 69, 70, 71
Rous, Sir Stanley, 133
Rowe, Iris, 17, 23

St Denis, Ruth, 50, 111, 159
Scott, Cyril, 25, 34
Seed, Audrey, 93
Segonzac, André de, 21
Sella, André, 44
Sella, Mr, 39, 40, 42
Shaw, George Bernard, 28
Shaw, Leila and Fred, 122
Shawn, Ted, 50, 111, 112,
    113, 115
Shelton, Brian, 120
Shone, Mrs, 46, 47
Shone, Norah, 11
Simpson, Betty, 54, 58, 79,
98, 102, 107, 121, 131, 134
Simpson, Dr, 54
Skinner, Jack, 88, 89, 93, 112,
    124
Spencer, Penelope, 23, 28
Stack, Prunella, 133
Steele, Tommy, 127
Stewart, John, 120
Stokes, Mildred, 24
Sykes, Mary, 65

Taylor, Willison, 102
Taylor-Elder, Andrew, 100, 102

Thorndike, Sybil, 28
Todd, Jane, 65
Tombazi, Mrs, 123
Tree, Viola, 11
Trevelyan, Sir Charles, 76
Tyrrell, Ann, 66, 67, 71, 76, 94
Tyrrell, Lord, 65, 66

Valois, Ninette de, 159, 162
Vanel, Hélène, 43

Wadsworth, Edward, 25
Watkinson, Kathleen, 229
Walter, Monica, 132
Wand-Tetley, Colonel, 88-91
Warre-Cornish, Gerald, 15
Warren, Lady, 123
Webster, Captain, A.M., 91
West, Barbara, 227
Whyte, Ian, 108, 124, 162
Wigman, Mary, 159
Wilkie, Miss, 77
Willert, Sir Arthur & Lady, 65, 66
Wills, Jan, 98
Windsor, Duke of, 44
Wolfit, Sir Donald, 28
Yarrow, Sir Harold & Lady, 123
Young, Anne, 126
Young, Professor A. McLaren, 27